Supporting Sick Children and their Families

To the nursing and medical staff in the Paediatric Intensive Care Unit and paediatric wards, and all those who contribute in so many ways towards the care of sick children at Addenbrooke's NHS Trust, Cambridge.

For Baillière Tindall:

Publishing Manager: Inta Ozols
Project Development Manager: Karen Gilmour
Project Manager: Derek Robertson

Supporting Sick Children and their Families

Penny Cook RSCN Cert.Couns.
Family Liaison Sister, Children's Services,
Addenbrooke's NHS Trust, Cambridge, UK

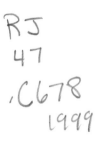

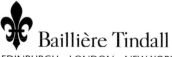 Baillière Tindall

EDINBURGH   LONDON   NEW YORK   PHILADELPHIA   ST LOUIS   SYDNEY   TORONTO 1999

BAILLIÈRE TINDALL
An imprint of Harcourt Publishers Limited

© Harcourt Publishers Limited 1999

✤ is a registered trademark of Harcourt Publishers Limited

First published 1999

ISBN 07020 22071

British Library Cataloguing in Publication Data
A catalogue record for this book is available from the British Library

Library of Congress Cataloging in Publication Data
A catalog record for this book is available from the Library of Congress

The
publisher's
policy is to use
**paper manufactured
from sustainable forests**

Printed in China

Contents

Acknowledgements

I have learnt an enormous amount from the families I have met over the years. I appreciate their honesty and willingness to share some of their deepest secrets, thoughts and feelings, sometimes during the worst moments of their lives. This gives me a feeling of enormous privilege and the insight to write about my experiences so that others may also learn. I have great admiration and respect for the courage and determination of so many unfortunate children and their families.

I am grateful to my own family for their encouragement and support, especially my husband Robert for his constant devotion and belief in me. I am quite sure that being married to me for thirty-something years he did not expect, or indeed deserve, to share the pressures of getting this book written.

I could not forget to thank all my friends and colleagues at Addenbrooke's Hospital, especially those who work for Childrens' Services. Their loyalty and trust in me has been rewarding, so I hope I have been able to help them and their patients. I am grateful to Rev. Ian Morris, hospital chaplain at Addenbrooke's, for kindly allowing me to publish his 'Five Ts of Bereavement First Aid'. I acknowledge Dr Glenys Parkinson, Chartered Psychologist, with thanks for her years of support and advice.

I appreciate the support of the team at Baillière Tindall, especially Sarah James for her enthusiasm with the initial suggestion of this book.

My thanks and good wishes to you all.

INTRODUCTION

I began my training as a Registered Sick Children's Nurse in 1961, at The Hospital for Sick Children, Great Ormond Street. The nurses wore starched aprons and caps and the young patients wore hospital clothes, many sewn or knitted by the dedicated army of volunteers who so faithfully supported the hospital. Parents were only allowed to visit their children at strictly designated times, and certainly not on the day of an operation. Much has changed since then, mostly for the better.

I had always wanted to be a nurse although I did not know much about what it would be like. My only experience of hospitals was having my wrist X-rayed or visiting someone on an 'adult' ward, and I remember the smell of disinfectant and unappetising food! I enjoyed being involved with children in a variety of ways, and so training as a children's nurse was an obvious progression from first aid monitor at school and child nurse badge in Guides.

It is helpful to look back occasionally, to see just how far we have come and what we have achieved. Learning from experience means utilising past experiences to gain new insights (Quinn, 1995). We must move with the times, taking our experiences with us, for as Jung (1933) commented: '*Today* stands between *yesterday* and *tomorrow* and forms a link between past and future, the present represents a process of transition'. The present is where we are *today* in this process of changing and evolving. Evolution is about the survival of the strongest or the best practice. Despite all the many changes in nursing, and in the health service as a whole, which have happened during recent years, the strongest and most basic elements of caring and compassion must survive.

Parents today play a full part in the care of their sick child, in partnership with the health professionals. The nurses share the care of children with their parents, exposing them all to scrutiny and criticism and increasing their need for support. Parents with a sick child are expected to be able to cope with extremes of physical and emotional endurance; brothers and sisters, and grandparents, have their own needs too.

The subsequent pressures on the family are not relieved by public perceptions and expectations, or by some misinformed journalists in the press and on television. It seems as if medical knowledge, surgical techniques and all the associated technology have advanced too rapidly for some members of the public to understand their implications and the high expectations they create. Time spent with parents to help them explore their own feelings and understanding is an essential part of caring for the family.

It is through working as a paediatric nurse, particularly in a paediatric intensive care unit, that I became aware of the huge range of emotions and feelings that arise for the patient, parents and family as well as for the staff. I value my experiences as a nurse and also as a wife, mother and grand-mother, and believe that by adding them to a counselling role I can offer a reasonable level of empathy and understanding.

I hope that this book is helpful for nurses, doctors, social workers, GPs, health visitors and students working with children, parents and siblings. Health professionals cannot work in isolation; they need good teamwork and understanding of what each role involves. They also need information about treatments and care given by others. Transplantation and organ donation are unfamiliar subjects unless you work in that specialised field, so I have included chapters on these. I hope that these will help staff at local hospitals or in the community to learn more about what their patients and their families have experienced.

This is not a pure textbook on nursing sick children, on bereavement or counselling – there are plenty of excellent books available, written in care-ful detail. It is not a book dictating what should be done, but I hope it will raise awareness of issues in order to help the reader choose what is right for each family and for the helper. I am a firm believer in responding to intuition – listening to yourself and doing what *feels* right – along with what you think and what you may be advised. Intuition must be reliable and trusted, and I believe it develops with the self-confidence of experience.

I have learnt much from children, their parents, families and friends, and the colleagues with whom I have worked. It is at times a great privi-lege and a humbling experience to be alongside people who share their deep personal and private thoughts with you, perhaps during a crisis when they are at their weakest and most vulnerable or at a very special or emotional time. I would like to think that my sense of being drained of energy means that they have gained some strength from the shared experience. I am grateful to all those who have trusted me, and thank them for what they have given me.

All the case studies in this book are real, from my own experience, with the names and situations altered to protect the identity of individuals.

This book is about what I have learnt, and I would like to pass it on to other health professionals. It has been written because I am asked to speak about my work, to spend time with students, to teach. I am not a teacher, but I am always happy to share my experiences with those who are interested to learn from what I have learnt. There is something rather special about handing on within a profession. This is how the apprentice learnt skills from the master craftsman; I hope that in this era of technology and emphasis on research-based learning, the human touch of personal experiences will not be lost.

> The teacher who walks in the shadow of the temple, among his followers, gives not of his wisdom but rather of his faith and his lovingness. If he is indeed wise he does not bid you enter the house of his wisdom, but rather leads you to the threshold of your own mind.
>
> (Gibran, 1926)

Medicine and nursing are often considered to be sciences, and indeed they are based on a scientific understanding – but they are also arts. The art of caring comes in the interpretation of facts and how we treat each individual child, parent, family or colleague. The same is true of counselling, which is both therapeutic and creative.

Caring for others, in whatever role that is, has often been referred to as a vocation or calling. I have mixed feelings about what that means, but I do know that it means a lot of learning, responsibility for our actions and to those we try to help, emotional and physical energy and dedication to the work. I remember carrying out a very important and sensitive task with a staff nurse I knew well. It was not easy or pleasant and she looked up and asked me: 'Why do I do this job?' She seemed to need an answer, and the only one that I could offer was: 'Because you can'. She often reminded me of this on later occasions – there was not really anything more to say, except that it is true that some people do jobs that others could not do.

My school motto was 'By love serve one another' (Galations, 5: 13) and I have to admit that, until relatively recently, I had not really considered what it meant. I now find it quite helpful, not as an order to serve others, but in its use of the word 'love' in the very broadest sense – the unconditional positive regard that Carl Rogers (1961) describes. The rather old-fashioned use of the word 'serve' suggests respect for others. This surely includes the five 'c's of caring identified by Roach (1987): compassion, competence, confidence, conscience and commitment.

I have written about some emotions and feelings, such as anger, fear, anxiety, guilt, responsibility, depression, loss and separation. I have given them their own chapters, although they are for consideration with the other chapter subjects. I believe that it is very important for health professionals to think about these words. How we act affects how we feel (behavioural theory) and how we think affects how we feel (cognitive theory). It will help to develop a better empathic understanding of what the family members are experiencing; it is too easy to label a parent as 'difficult'.

Working alongside people who are experiencing an unbearable period in their lives can be desperately hard and these caring people need support too. Sometimes it is helpful to think of problems through images or illustrations, and following is one I have offered to people in particularly difficult times. Think about a boat, perhaps a fishing boat, out at sea when a storm blows up. The boat is too small to stand up to the rough sea and gales; it would not survive. The skipper steers the boat closer to the shore, to the shelter of a bay with protection from the cliffs. He drops the anchor for security and although the boat may still swing freely with the tide and the waves, it will not drift away. The crew members ride out the storm by making the boat as safe as possible, staying still and only doing what is essential. Those who help people in stormy periods of their lives are providing the shelter from the storm; the anchor which secures, yet allows freedom. They cannot take away the storm, but can perhaps aim to make it more bearable while waiting for the calm.

Penny Cook
Cambridge, 1999

REFERENCES

Galations, 5 v13. The New Testament, Holy Bible.

Gibran, K (1926) *The Prophet*. London: Heinemann.

Jung, C. (1933) *Modern Man in Search of a Soul*. London: Ark Paperbacks, Routledge

Quinn, F. (1995) *Principles and Practice of Nurse Education*.Cheltenham: Stanley Thornes.

Roach, M.S. (ed) (1987) *The Human Act of Caring*. Ottowa: Canadian Hospital Association.

Rogers, C. (1961) *On Becoming a Person*. London: Constable.

Support

INTRODUCTION

Support is a word used quite frequently in the context of sickness, hospitals, emergencies and traumatic events, but do we always know what we, or others, mean by it? When we look in the dictionary we find many definitions of the word, and it is interesting to consider how very appropriate most of them are to our study of sick children and their families. The *Concise Oxford Dictionary* (1990) offers the following definitions:

1. Carry all or part of the weight of
2. keep from falling or sinking or failing
3. provide with a home and the necessities of life
4. enable to last out; give strength to; encourage
5. bear out; tend to substantiate or corroborate
6. give help or countenance to, back up; second, further
7. speak in favour of
8. be actively interested in
9. take a part that is secondary to
10. assist by one's presence
11. endure, tolerate
12. maintain or represent adequately
13. subscribe to the funds of.

It would perhaps be helpful to use these as a guide to explore our understanding of support and, alongside this, to ask the question: 'Who needs support?'.

Throughout this book, the different people involved will be considered in terms of the groups defined in Box 1.1.

Box 1.1 Groups involved in the care of sick children

- Children
- Parents
- Brothers and sisters
- Grandparents
- Child's friends

- Professionals
  - — hospital nurses and doctors
  - — community nurses, health visitors
  - — general practitioners
  - — school teachers, school nurse

THE DEFINITIONS OF SUPPORT

'Carry all or part of the weight of'

Illness brings with it many burdens for families to carry, and it is usually helpful if other people can relieve them of some of the weight, to make these burdens more bearable. If a child requires admission to hospital in an emergency, it is a great relief to the parents to know that their other child (or children) is being well cared for by a relative or friend, so that they do not have to worry about that child as well.

Parents of a child with a chronic condition or disability may become desperate for respite care. This could involve help for a few hours a week to enable the mother to go shopping without having to take a wheelchair, time to give undivided attention to another child, time to spend with her partner or friends, or time for herself to read or even just sleep. In some areas, a service is available offering experienced babysitters – often nurses, nursery nurses or mothers of older children.

It makes a great difference to one parent to have good support from the other; there is a fairly basic need to share decisions and responsibilities with the other person who should have the child's best interests in mind (see Case Study 1.1). Mothers usually stay in hospital, but there are many reasons why a father may be the one to do this; sometimes the father is the child's main carer. He, too, may or may not have the support of the child's mother or of a partner. It is important to support the parents' partnership by encouraging mutual respect in a teamwork approach. This may include help with planning and sharing of the tasks to be covered, such as who will stay in hospital each night, who will care for any children at home or which parent could continue to work (even if only part-time).

It is important for parents to be able to share their concerns with the medical and nursing staff, and to be certain that they have all the relevant information required to make informed

---

CASE STUDY 1.1 *Taking responsibility alone*

Tracey was a single mother; the father of her son had left soon after the baby was born. When her child was 6 years old, he needed major surgery, and although Tracey had a few months to prepare for this, it was a terrible ordeal for her. The hardest stage for her was signing the consent form for the operation – there was no-one to share the weight of this responsibility. After the child was safely in the operating theatre, she was shaking, saying she wished she had a husband to share this. She carried a heavy burden of guilt for a long time.

decisions. This helps them to feel that others are sharing some of the weight of decision-making.

Talking with other parents can also relieve some of the burden. Parents with children of similar ages or with similar symptoms, or who are simply in hospital at the same time, are often able to share feelings and ways of coping. There are now a great number of support organisations for most children's conditions, and families can gain specialist information and advice as well as simply being able to contact other families who are, or who have experienced, living with children with particular problems.

'Keep from falling or sinking or failing'

A mother once described in detail how she felt as though she were on the edge of a high cliff; she could not bear to look over the edge in case she fell. Her child was critically ill and she was afraid that she was at the limits of her stamina. She could not go back as she needed to be with her child, in the present, and she could not look ahead as the future was uncertain. Her great concern was that she should not fall or sink lest she fail her child.

Parents, particularly mothers, have a fear of failing their children and may need considerable reassurance to remind them that they are doing all they can for their child. There may be times when they need holding, in the same way that they are holding the child. There are many occasions when a helping hand, an arm to lean on or a shoulder to cry on really does prevent someone in distress from falling. Talking through problems usually helps, and a counselling approach would encourage a person to find her own inner strengths and the ability to hold on.

'Provide with a home and the necessities of life'

Whatever the family situation or wherever they are, a family needs somewhere to call home. They also need food, clothes and sleep. Most hospitals caring for sick children provide accommodation for a parent to stay with a child and should have facilities for parents to eat and take a break away from the ward.

Parents not in permanent employment, and those who are self-employed and unable to work because of the sick child may get into financial difficulties. Those who are eligible receive the relevant benefits and assistance from social security. Social workers and advice centres are useful sources of advice on these matters.

The sick child needs the security of knowing that even in hospital, a temporary home can be safe and will provide what is needed. Places to play, to keep personal possessions, to watch favourite television programmes and videos and to provide some privacy for older children are all important considerations.

'Enable to last out; give strength to; encourage'

This definition of support has a more desperate feel to it, but there are times when it is applicable. When a child is critically ill, members of the family do feel desperate; they are afraid, tired and confused, and they cling on to any hope that can be offered. Hope is what gives them strength and encouragement, and somehow they are able to keep on going for the child's sake.

Often, when people feel desperate and need to find strength from somewhere, they find it spiritually, either in their own way or with a minister of their religion. If the hospital chapel is open at all times, it offers a quiet place to be alone for prayers or with private thoughts. Most hospitals have a chaplain available and the family's own minister would be welcome.

Parents often have a fear of not lasting out for the child's sake; sometimes it is helpful for them to sit down quietly and go over what has happened, to acknowledge how hard it has been and to recognize that they have survived until now and can survive longer. There may be strong feelings from the parents, encouraging the child to be strong. I have watched mothers holding the hands of unconscious children willing their own strength to pass to the child.

'Bear out; tend to substantiate or corroborate'

This might be about professionals working together as a well-informed team in partnership with parents, bearing out what has been learnt concerning the child's condition. Parents should be able to ask questions and to give and be given appropriate and honest information that may substantiate a diagnosis. It is also about effective communication between family members including the child. Parents describe symptoms to the doctor, bearing out what the child has said.

'Give help or countenance to, back up, second, further'

Care from health professionals, especially in hospitals, is continuous. This means that there is much 'handing over' – at the end of nursing shifts, to doctors on call, at weekends, during periods of staff sickness etc. It seems like a constant back-up system and each handover has to take the patient and family further in the care process.

It is understandable that when parents are given a diagnosis for their child, they will want to be certain that it is correct. They may ask for further information, seek a second opinion from a different doctor and discuss with the nurses the implications of what they have been told. Of all the definitions, this one, of 'giving help', is the most fundamental.

'Speak in favour of'

Health professionals should always be speaking in favour of their patients and families. On ward rounds and at team meetings, the family's thoughts and requests should be part of the discussions. In paediatrics we must always be aware of being the child's advocate, especially when the parents are unable to perform this role. The nurse who is looking after a child may be the right person to speak on his behalf when a particular procedure is suggested. Issues surrounding the child's fear or understanding and feeling of pain are common examples.

'Be actively interested in'

It makes an enormous difference to how the parents view the medical and nursing staff if they feel that the staff are really interested in their child and their family. If a surgeon does not make a point of seeing the parents after operating on a child or if a nurse does not discuss the child's care, the parents may lose trust in them and feel that nobody cares. The danger then is that this vital trust cannot be regained.

The skills of listening attentively, allowing the speaker to communicate what they really need to say or ask, are fundamentally important. Needless to say, having a conversation whilst reading, writing, answering the bleep or telephone or looking out of the window is not advisable. It is often helpful to reflect back what has been said by the other party and to indicate that you have remembered the important facts.

'Take a part that is secondary to'

One way of understanding this type of support is to think of supporting actors playing a secondary role to the principals. They are not the stars of the show but are essential to the production. The same is true in health care teams, where all roles, both principal and supporting, are important in the delivery of suitable care.

We should remember that parents are normally the prime carers for a child and that any involved professionals, be they medical or nursing staff, social workers, teachers or childminders, are all secondary to the parents. The children do not belong to us; they belong with their parents and their family.

'Assist by one's presence'

An experienced nurse can provide support to a more junior nurse by being present while the latter carries out a procedure. This can help to build confidence and ensure safe practice. Similarly, when important information or bad news has to be given to parents, doctors often find it helpful if a nurse is present, as do the parents themselves who are likely to have developed a trusting relationship with the nurse. As a listener and observer, the nurse will be able to watch the parents' reactions and perhaps interpret medical information or repeat it later.

Friends and relations of a sick child often visit the family, in hospital or at home, because they would like to be supportive to them. There may be very little they can do to help, but by making the effort to visit they show they care.

'Endure, tolerate'

Sometimes, when life seems particularly tough and there is not much chance of an early improvement in the situation, surviving may feel more like an endurance test. The parents usually endure or tolerate for the sake of their child: 'I don't like what is happening, but while he is ill I will put up with difficulties for him.'

'Maintain or represent adequately'

Parents play a key role in maintaining their sick child: they keep the child clean and clothed, fed and cared for. Hospital staff also have a maintenance role. For example, dieticians talk about maintenance nutrition and fluids, while physiotherapists maintain the body's ability to move and the lungs' ability to expand properly. Social workers may help to maintain the family's ability to cope with a child's illness or condition by advising on benefits, housing or child care during a difficult time.

'Subscribe to the funds of'

Everyone who has a taxable financial income subscribes to the funds of the National Health Service, the social services and the community services and in this sense they are providing support. In addition there are many people who contribute to voluntary organisations working for particular causes. Many families and their friends raise money for special equipment to help a child at home or at a school for children with special needs. A large amount of expensive equipment in intensive care units and children's wards is donated by grateful families after their child is better, or given in memory of a child who died.

The number of support organisations for particular conditions continues to grow, and clearly they fulfil a valuable role in advising and supporting families. They are usually run as charities and depend on donations for their income

SEEKING SOCIAL SUPPORT

Carver Scheier and Weintraub (1989), in a lengthy study of coping strategies, found seeking social support for instrumental and emotional reasons to be an important strategy (see Box 1.2). The examples in Box 1.2 highlight the value of finding the right information and of talking to people who may help. Those working in any of the 'caring' professions will know that one important line of support is access to good, honest and appropriate information.

Talking to a trusted person usually helps; this might be a friend or relative, a member of the health care team or someone who has had a similar experience. Parents often talk to other parents with children in the same hospital or clinic. In this way they can

---

Box 1.2 Seeking social support (Carver et al., 1989)

For instrumental reasons:
- 'I ask people who have had similar experiences what they did.'
- 'I try to get advice from someone about what to do.'
- 'I talk to someone to find out more about the situation.'
- 'I talk to someone who could do something concrete about the problem'

For emotional reasons:
- 'I talk to someone about how I feel.'
- 'I try to get emotional support from friends or relatives.'
- 'I discuss my feelings with someone.'
- 'I get sympathy and understanding from someone.'

share their problems, and perhaps off-load some of their anxiety, as well as helping each other with alternative suggestions and ideas.

Sick children need good support which should be tailored to their age and state of health. Having appropriate information and the opportunity to talk helps them to be prepared, so that they know what to expect and do not feel isolated during anxious and uncertain periods. Play specialists help younger children to communicate through play, drawing and acting.

PARENT SUPPORT GROUPS

Many parents find support groups helpful as a safe forum for sharing and learning from others' experiences. Some groups are held in a hospital setting, perhaps on a ward for children with similar medical conditions. A nurse with a good knowledge of the medical facts and treatments may facilitate such a group and it will often become a helpful resource for information and reassurance. Counsellors, social workers or chaplains may also facilitate support groups like these.

Other groups, such as those for bereaved parents, may be held away from familiar hospital areas, and parents find great comfort in sharing their feelings with others who know and understand (see Ch. 15).

Many families receive helpful information and advice from the various national support groups which exist for most congenital and chronic conditions and syndromes. Some have local branches or newsletters as a way of keeping in contact with other parents and all give contact telephone numbers so that parents of children with similar problems can talk to each other. A comprehensive directory, which is updated regularly, is published by Contact-a-Family (1998).

TEAMWORK

Teamwork is so important that it deserves to be mentioned again. A team whose members are working well together will provide support both for the individual team members and for the team as a whole in partnership with the family. This in turn enables family members to do what is best for the child and for themselves.

Caring for sick children is often stressful and health professionals need to know where they can find helpful support for themselves. Some find it useful to have regular team meetings to discuss difficult issues and the thoughts and feelings that result.

Employing authorities should establish training and support provision for staff involved in helping a family to care for a child with a life-limiting incurable disease (While *et al.*, 1996).

In this context of supporting sick children and their families, there are many 'teams', each as important as the other:

- the sick child within the family
- the family in partnership with the professionals and other carers
- the child and the health care team.

CONCLUSION

We can see that there are many ways of understanding support, all of them relevant in some way to the sick child, the family and others involved with the care. The underlying aim is to enable people to help themselves to survive a period of crisis or long-term problems or to come to terms with the difficult situation in which they find themselves. Perhaps after exploring various aspects of support, the essential benefits may be realised, and the value of sharing and working together appreciated.

REFERENCES

Carver, C., Scheier, M. & Weintraub, J. (1989) 'Assessing coping strategies: a theoretically based approach. *Journal of Personality and Social Psychology,* **56,** 267–283.

Contact-a-Family (1998) *Directory of Specific Conditions and Rare Syndromes in Children with their Family Support Networks,* 2nd edn (with six-monthly updates). London: Contact-a-Family.

While, A., Citrone, C. & Cornish, J. (1996) *A Study of the Needs and Provisions for Families Caring for Children with Life-limiting Incurable Disorders.* King's College, London: Department of Nursing Studies.

Defence mechanisms and coping strategies

INTRODUCTION

Defences are a natural and necessary protection against painful and seemingly unbearable events; we all use them at times to help us through threatening circumstances. They may help our survival in times of danger, and if we are preoccupied with taking avoiding action we become less aware of the intense anxiety. For anxious parents whose child is sick, their defence mechanisms come into play as part of their way of coping with a dreadful situation.

From my own observations, I have found that many parents have difficulty managing the fine balance between survival through protection by some form of defence and coping with facing the harsh truth. This is hardly surprising and calls for considerable awareness and teamwork amongst the carers, especially when giving important and potentially devastating information.

An important element in the teamwork is a shared understanding of the ways in which the child and the family members are dealing with the situation. When a child is critically ill, family members may need to change their thinking frequently, as the child's condition may change from hour to hour. For parents of a child with a long-term or even lifetime illness or disability, it is useful to have regular assessments of how they are coping with their circumstances. When parents appear to be coping well, health professionals sometimes neglect to offer them the opportunity to talk about the things that are really important to them, and these assessments allow them to air their concerns.

Parents can all too readily be labelled as 'awkward' or 'difficult' and an essential part of the caring role is to try to understand the feelings and emotions behind the words and actions. Professionals using good counselling skills need to work at helping parents to recognise and acknowledge their own defences, rather than criticising them, and to understand them. With this recognition and understanding, parents can more easily move forwards to recognising their own strengths and weaknesses, thus enabling them to cope better with their situation.

Carl Rogers (1961) defined the opposite of defensiveness as 'being open to experience'. His style of person-centred therapy aims to help individuals to become more openly aware of their own attitudes and feelings – 'not a facade of conformity to others, not a cynical denial of all feeling, nor a front of intellectual rationality'. There is also a message here for the professionals who care for sick children and their families.

Freud (1894) first thought that defence caused anxiety, but later changed his mind, believing that defence was, in fact, provoked by anxiety. His theories about anxiety and defence arose from his observations of neurotic conditions such as hysteria. He later referred to this particular defence as 'repression', and went on to describe others. For the family of a very sick child, anxiety is a reaction to the threat of loss. The loss may not be total, as in death, but could be the loss of what is normal for that family, and loss of future hopes and aspirations. This must be recognised and acknowledged by the staff caring for the family, and some understanding of how the defences are put into play is of considerable importance in the supportive counselling role.

This chapter explores some of the defence mechanisms and strategies for coping used by families with a sick child.

DENIAL

When our outside world becomes too threatening, our egos shut off the painful experiences by denial, i.e. we deny 'the perceptions that would involve acknowledging the reality of the situation' (Nelson-Jones, 1982).

It is well known that someone who is responsible for an accident may deny all knowledge of it and be unable to recall any of the events associated with it. Likewise, patients needing an operation may say they have no pain or symptoms, thus pretending that they do not have a problem. Our paediatric patients often choose not to talk about an imminent procedure because they are denying their fears. Denial of this type is a recognised means of coping in children (Eiser, 1990).

If parents are trying to deny the truth of their child's condition, they may be forcing themselves to have hope. Well-meaning relatives have perhaps used the old saying 'where there's life there's hope'. Health professionals must be careful when giving information to be honest so that they do not build false hopes, and yet it is important not to destroy all hope. Consistent and appropriate answers from medical and nursing staff will be supportive in allowing a gradual acceptance of the situation.

Judd (1989), a child psychotherapist working with children with life-threatening and terminal illnesses and their families, wrote:

If defences enable the child and his parents to carry on living without unbearable degrees of anxiety, then they are effective and useful (Chodoff *et al.*, 1964). However, if the defences lead to family members being locked in a web of silence, unable to talk to each other for fear of breakdown, this adds to the stress and anxiety of each individual (Turk, 1964). They may continue to function without breakdown, but at considerable psychological cost.

Judd recognised that some degree of denial can be a useful defence, but that it can have disastrous results if the silence and pretence are allowed to continue for too long. Every opportunity should be offered for talking about the situation, in order to address the issues with someone who is able to listen without finding it unbearable. Nobody is going to burden another person, especially someone in the family, with their pain of the truth if that person does not appear able to understand or accept what is being said.

Spufford (1989), writing about her experiences in hospitals with her child, stated:

I have listened to people who were similarly failing to face the actual difficulties that presented themselves. They too were trying to persuade themselves that other people's circumstances were more difficult.

The nurse or other carer for a child will usually observe how each individual parent is dealing with the situation. Quite often, one parent is being realistic while the other is denying the truth and being inappropriately optimistic (see Case Study 2.1).

CASE STUDY 2.1   *Acceptance by one parent; denial by the other*

Michael's parents were in a room with the consultant and a nurse to be given the result of their son's brain scan. After a careful explanation of the facts the doctor told them that their son could not survive. His mother sat back in her chair and said simply, 'I knew that's what you were going to say. I have known deep down, ever since the accident, that we were going to lose him, but I had hoped it would not be true.' At this her husband looked at her in utter amazement; he appeared so shocked he could not speak. He had refused to think of anything other than a complete recovery, and was surprised at his wife's comment. A little later he was able to admit that he had totally denied the truth because he did not want to face it.

THE VALUE OF HOPE

We need to remember that hope is what keeps people going. If there is no light at the end of the proverbial tunnel, it is hard to imagine an end or a resolution of the problem. Parents often seem to deny the signs of a child's condition, especially if it could be life-threatening or life-limiting. They are hoping against hope that the diagnosis is not correct – of course they do not want it to be true (see Case Study 2.2).

CASE STUDY 2.2   Coping by deferring the truth

The mother of a baby born with Down's syndrome could not accept the diagnosis for several days. She would say that she thought her baby looked perfectly normal and would stroke the little hands and feet. Gradually, she was able to move on to see that her baby did look slightly different from the other babies, and she started to ask questions about the condition and learn about local support.

I have seen nurses who were greatly concerned that a mother appeared to remain cheerful when her child was critically ill. Their concern was that the mother did not fully understand the severity of the situation; otherwise she would not be so cheerful. I sensed that the nurses were not comfortable with the mother's cheery nature. But would they have found it easier if the mother was constantly tearful or angry? My own feelings are that we do not have the right to remove a mother's (or father's) remaining defence at this juncture and that we should support her in the way she chooses to behave, but in the knowledge that she really does understand the situation.

In one case like this, I spoke about it with the mother and discovered that, in fact, she was being remarkably strong. She was under no illusions as to the possible sad outcome of the child's condition, and said it was something with which she had lived for most of the child's life. She felt safe and cared for in the intensive care unit because she knew that everyone understood what was happening to her and felt she did not have to say anything. She just wanted to be with her child, knowing that everything possible was being done. She did not feel as safe outside and could not cope with meeting people who tried to be sympathetic, so she chose with care the visitors with whom she was happy to go out for lunch or tea. In this case, a nurse was present when the consultant discussed the child's poor prognosis and possible death with the mother, and so witnessed what was said between them. This team understanding is highly important, and it may have helped the nurses to understand the mother's quiet, fairly cheerful attitude.

Unless acknowledgement and expression of good and bad feelings are allowed and encouraged, there could be a strengthening of resistance on the part of a parent, which later becomes a barrier to realistic appreciation of the situation.

DEFENCE MECHANISMS

Sigmund Freud's daughter, Anna, identified 12 mechanisms of defence (Freud, 1936; Brown and Pedder, 1979) (see Box 2.1). In addition, Melaine Klein identified the mechanisms of 'splitting' and 'projective identification' (Box 2.1).

Box 2.1 Mechanisms of defence	
• Regression	• Turning against the self
• Repression	• Reversal
• Reaction formation	• Sublimation
• Isolation	• Idealisation
• Undoing	• Identification with the aggressor
• Projection	• Splitting
• Introjection	• Projective identification

Below, I will discuss some of these mechanisms in the context of my own observations of families in hospital.

Regression

Regression is used to describe a return to an earlier stage in one's development or a 'safer' time in life. When we become ill and in need of medical or nursing help, we often regress to some earlier degree of dependence. We may have to accept advice from a professional 'father' or dominant 'mother' figure in the doctor and quite easily adopt a temporary child-like response to the nurturing and parenting role of the nurse. Berne (1964) discussed the parent–adult–child ego states in his 'transactional analysis'. He regarded the unit of social intercourse as a transaction. The analysis of the transaction is concerned with which ego state implemented the transactional stimulus and which ego state executed the transactional response.

One can see how this applies to a sick child's parents as they seek leadership from those in some role of authority – other adults who can be trusted with the responsibility. They ask permission to touch their own child for fear of unknowingly dislodging a drainage tube or intravenous line. They are acutely aware of their inadequate skills, which adds to their feeling of helplessness in the situation. They may need careful encouragement to take even a small part in the child's care, at least until there is sufficient improvement to give them some hope of a normal recovery.

The child's grandparents sometimes play a considerable role as they resume their own parenting skills. It is not unusual for a young mother to admit that she needs her own mother at this time, and may desperately need a hug. A grandmother may respond by coming in to help with other children in the family, doing the shopping and washing, and providing meals. By helping in the home she is giving valuable practical assistance to the parents and child in hospital.

The emotional needs of grandparents should also be recognised. They too have regressed, to a lesser extent, into the earlier parenting role. It may be important to give them time to talk; they may be suffering themselves as they remember their time as young parents. I once felt the deep pain of a grandmother as she told me about the death in hospital of a child of hers, at the same age as her daughter's child who was now ill. She was reliving the horrors and grieving, and needed to express her own feelings in order to be able to support her daughter.

Sick children may regress because they are physically unable to maintain their independence and earlier levels of achievement. They may also find comfort and reassurance from extra attention when they feel particularly insecure and afraid.

It is not unusual for the brothers and sisters of a sick child to show signs of regression. They may cling to their parents and show distress when being left with friends during visits to hospital, when they would normally stay happily with them. Refusing to attend school or eat normal meals, wetting the bed when usually dry at night, thumb sucking and baby talk are also recognisable signs of regression in children with underlying anxiety. The parents may benefit from some reassurance, as these new problems could add to an increasing sense of guilt (feeling they have failed their children), anger and confusion.

Suppression and repression

Uncomfortable feelings of anxiety, fear or anger are often suppressed if there is no suitable way of dealing with them, or if the person cannot handle them. However, although they may be out of sight, the person will usually be aware of their existence, just below the surface, and sometimes they will reappear when it is least convenient or appropriate.

It is possible for unbearable feelings to be suppressed to such an extent that the person may withdraw into a passive state of indecision and acceptance as a response to the threats. Psychosomatic symptoms may result from suppressing bad feelings for too long – headaches, insomnia, joint pains, diarrhoea and nausea are not uncommon.

In repression, conscious thoughts and memories are pushed into the unconscious as if to banish them from access. Nelson-Jones (1982) commented that 'repression is the central underlying defensive mechanism of the ego, the basis of all other defences'. In counselling, the client is enabled to return to these issues in order to resolve them and rebuild on a more secure foundation of experience.

Projection

Bad feelings, particularly about ourselves, are sometimes not acceptable to us, and thoughts and feelings will be described as if they have come from another person. The need to dissociate ourselves from these thoughts and to ascribe them to someone else can result in a feeling that the rest of the world is hostile. This is sometimes seen when parents complain about traits in others which are visible in the parents themselves. Similarly, parents with desperate hopes for their child's recovery may project the necessary skills onto the doctors and nurses caring for her, and will praise them excessively.

Splitting

In splitting, good and bad thoughts and aspects of one's own and other people's personalities are split off and separated. This is an unhelpful and potentially destructive simplification of reality and we have to be careful not to encourage parents to split the health care system into 'good' and 'bad' doctors, and 'good' and 'bad' hospitals.

Idealisation

When 'good' and 'bad' have been split, it can lead on to the good person being regarded as perfect or ideal. Any other attributes displayed by this person that do not fit this picture are ignored. This is usually unrealistic and can lead to a loss of self-esteem and depression. If a parent or a child idealises a particular nurse, doctor, hospital, ward or treatment as being wonderful and all others as not so good, it makes treating that child difficult. The patient may need to be admitted or have treatment at a time when a different person is working, or in a different place.

Turning against the self

This generally happens when people take the blame for events beyond their control, and direct their anger and frustration inwards. They have a poor self-image and a strong sense of worthlessness. This is sometimes seen in parents who are feeling that they have let their child down. Self-harm and even suicide attempts are ways of turning anger against the self. At the same time, others are hurt and are made to feel guilty (Jacobs, 1982), which can provide a sense of much-needed satisfaction.

Displacement

Displacement describes the process of a dream image representing something else, or one activity substituting for another. In cases of displacement, feelings and impulses are redirected from one person or object to another.

On one occasion, a father became very angry because his child had suffered another setback in recovery from a major operation. He would not listen to reasonable information which should have helped him to understand the child's problems. On his way out of the ward, he punched his fist through the glass panel of the door. He cut his hand and of course there was a dangerous scattering of glass. It is possible that he was redirecting the urge to hit the doctor who gave him the 'bad news' or even his child for not getting better when he could not cope any more.

Isolation

Rycroft (1968) defined isolation as: 'a defence mechanism by which the subject isolates an occurrence, preventing it from becoming part of the continuum of his significant experience'. Thus, an unpleasant experience is not allowed to have any effect on or connection with other events. Parents, and families as a whole, may choose to isolate themselves by not mixing with other parents and by not keeping in touch with family and friends by telephone. They feel more secure by withdrawing to a safe place where they do not have to talk to other people. It is not uncommon for a parent to stay out of sight when doctors come round, imagining: 'If I am not there they can't tell me bad news.'

This has been a brief discussion of the complex subject of defence mechanisms. Most defences are ways of trying to cope with thoughts, feelings or memories that are too threatening to admit fully into consciousness (Jacobs, 1982). Those of us working with families in difficult situations need to be able to recognise these defences in the resistance we encounter. We may need to go along with them for a while until the person is more capable of emerging from behind the protective barrier of defence.

COPING STRATEGIES

I would like to begin by asking the question: 'What is coping, and what do we mean by coping?' The *Concise Oxford Dictionary* (1990) defines 'cope' as: 'deal effectively or contend successfully with a person or task; deal with a situation or problem'. Sick children and their families and friends have to 'deal' with many people and tasks, situations and problems. The aim is to be able to survive a difficult period successfully.

There does seem to be a fear of not being able to cope. Parents often say, 'I don't know how I am going to cope.' One mother said to me that she did so want to cope because she could not bear pathetic women. Jennings (1992a) showed that, of all the problems faced by mothers of sick children, coping was the greatest.

Just as we develop ways of defending ourselves from unbearable thoughts and events, so we develop ways of coping with stressful situations. Much of how we do this is dependent on our individual personalities, on how we respond to changes and unpredictable events in life and on whether there is any time to prepare. Previous experiences play an important part in this, as well as the opportunity to talk to someone else who has been through a similar experience.

Research into coping with stress has been going on for many years. Lazarus (1966) suggested that stress consists of three processes:

- *primary appraisal* – the process of perceiving a threat to oneself
- *secondary appraisal* – the process of bringing to mind a potential response to the threat
- *coping* – the process of executing that response.

Lazarus (1974) also identified two types of coping – defensive and direct – while Jennings (1992a) later suggested that coping may be described from both a psychological and a sociological viewpoint.

In the early to mid-1980s a 'Ways of Coping Scale' was developed by Folkman and Lazarus (1980, 1985), and later, Carver *et al.*(1989) described two general types of coping:

- problem-focused coping – aimed at problem-solving or doing something to alter the source of the stress
- emotion-focused coping – aimed at reducing or managing the emotional distress that is associated with the situation.

Montagne and Pawlak (1990) used the Ways of Coping Scale in a study of parents coping with a child in intensive care. They found that two strategies were used most frequently in dealing with the predominant stressor: *seeking social support* (problem-focused mode) and *positive reappraisal* (emotion-focused mode). Overall, the parents used slightly more emotion-focused coping than problem-focused coping: 56 vs. 44%.

Carver *et al.* (1989) listed 14 coping strategies in a detailed study of how individuals respond to stressful events in their lives. These are detailed in Box 2.2, along with examples of each.

Box 2.2 Coping strategies in response to stressful events (Carver *et al.*, 1989).

Active coping
- I take additional action to get rid of the problem
- I concentrate my efforts on doing something about it
- I do what has to be done, one step at a time
- I take direct action to get around the problem

Planning
- I try to come up with a strategy about what to do
- I make a plan of action
- I think hard about what steps to take
- I think about how I might best handle the problem

Suppression of competing activities
- I put aside other activities in order to concentrate on this
- I focus on dealing with this problem, and if necessary, let other things slide a little
- I keep myself from getting distracted by other thoughts or activities
- I try hard to prevent other things from interfering with my efforts at dealing with this

Restrained coping
- I force myself to wait for the right time to do something
- I hold off doing anything about it until the situation permits
- I make sure not to make matters worse by acting too soon
- I restrain myself from doing anything too quickly

Seeking social support for instrumental reasons
- I ask people who have had similar experiences what they did
- I try to get advice from someone about what to do
- I talk to someone to find out more about the situation
- I talk to someone who could do something concrete about the problem

Seeking social support for emotional reasons
- I talk to someone about how I feel
- I try to get emotional support from friends or relatives
- I discuss my feelings with someone
- I get sympathy and understanding from someone

Positive reinterpretation and growth
- I look for something good in what is happening
- I try to see it in a different light, to make it seem more positive
- I learn something from the experience
- I try to grow as a person as a result of the experience

Acceptance
- I learn to live with it
- I accept that this has happened and that it cannot be changed
- I get used to the idea that it happened
- I accept the reality of the fact that it happened

Turning to religion
- I seek God's help
- I put my trust in God
- I try to find comfort in my religion
- I pray more than usual

Focus and venting of emotions
- I get upset and let my emotions out
- I let my feelings out
- I feel a lot of emotional distress and find myself expressing those feelings a lot
- I get upset, and I am really aware of it

Denial
- I refuse to believe that it has happened
- I pretend that it hasn't really happened
- I act as though it hasn't even happened
- I say to myself 'this isn't real'

Behavioural disengagement
- I give up the attempt to get what I want
- I just give up trying to reach my goal
- I admit to myself that I can't deal with it, and quit trying
- I reduce the amount of effort I'm putting into solving the problem

Mental disengagement
- I turn to work or other substitute activities to take my mind off things
- I go to movies or watch TV, to think about it less
- I daydream about things other than this
- I sleep more than usual

Alcohol–drug disengagement
- I drink alcohol or take drugs, in order to think about it less

A study of parents of children who received liver transplants (Noble-Jamieson *et al.*, 1996) identified the major stress factors and parental coping strategies before transplantation, during the hospital admission and after the child's discharge. In addition to the coping techniques listed in Box 2.2 the parents described the following:

- being unrealistic,
- being realistic
- rationalisations
- anticipation of a problem
- passive awaiting – 'I have no control'
- making others or circumstances responsible
- trust
- ability to let go
- escape into illness (psychosomatic symptoms)
- rigid belief system.

The most frequently used coping strategies in each phase were: 'being realistic', 'having trust in the medical team' and 'accepting the situation'. At all stages parents wanted, and were given, time to talk to the medical team to seek more information. Emotional support from relatives and friends was valuable for sympathy and understanding.

In order for parents to be realistic, appropriate truthful information must be given to and understood by them, and adequate time offered for them to ask questions. A study of a number of mothers in hospital with their children (Schepp, 1991) concluded that 'mothers who knew what events to expect experienced less anxiety and reported expending less effort to cope with the stressful events'. Schepp reported on several studies which showed that the more information the parents had about their ill child's condition, the less anxiety they experienced.

Trust in the medical team and the nursing staff is an essential requirement for successful coping; this may take time to develop, and honesty will be an important factor (see Case Study 2.3).

CASE STUDY 2.3   The importance of honesty

Ann's mother was shaking with shock when the hospital doctor explained that her daughter would not be able to survive her sudden severe illness. She begged him to keep trying to save her, and the doctor gently repeated the facts, honestly but simply.

Later in the day, the mother asked to see the doctor to thank him for being so honest from the time Ann was admitted. She said she was only able to cope with the rest of the awful day because everyone had been truthful with her.

Coping by fathers

It is not unusual for fathers to distance themselves from the sick child, often using work commitments as the reason for this. I have known fathers who put so much energy into work at a time when the family was under great strain that they have not been able to keep this going. A mental breakdown, physical illness or loss of employment has been the result.

Lansky (1974) wrote of this tendency for fathers to abandon the family psychologically during serious illness, by spending increased amounts of time away from home, and stated: 'The more a father is separated from the situation ... where the mother may shut him out emotionally, the more a father may feel jealous, threatened, and certainly unprepared for a possible death'.

Practical help

For some family situations, a little extra help with practical issues may make a big difference to how the family copes. Some mothers become very organised and make arrangements for who will meet other children from school, help with shopping and hospital visits. If grandparents live near enough, they may be able to help; indeed, doing something useful for the family may help *them* to cope with the anxiety. It may be possible for a social worker or community nurse to arrange for respite care, help at home, or a nursery place for a sibling. If some of the practical and domestic problems can be eased, then the pressure on the family is not quite so overwhelming and the parents have a better chance of coping with the emotional stress.

Planning ahead

Many parents cope by planning ahead whenever possible, so information and possible time-scales are important (see Case Study 2.4).

CASE STUDY 2.4

Parents caring for their child at home with a terminal condition were anxious when the child became weaker and needing nasogastric tube feeds. This was a significant stage in the child's deteriorating state of health and was quite a hurdle in their acceptance of the situation. Time was given, away from home, to explore the parents' fears of how they would manage to nurse their child and how they would cope with her death at home. When it happened, they were very capable and calm.

By thinking ahead and addressing the possible and probable events and using phrases and words associated with what would happen, the fears became less frightening and their confidence in their own ability was strengthened.

Coping by children

Children are usually dependent on their parents for help in coping with their illness, disability and treatment, and so the way the parents cope will affect a child's ability to cope. It is sensible to help the parents to help the child, taking into account the child's age, earlier experiences, personality and family dynamics. As already discussed, children will defend themselves by using denial and pretence, and often need to be encouraged by adults to talk about their illness or other problems.

Children can be taught techniques for coping with pain and procedures such as injections. Allowing children to have some control over events, for example in the management of an asthmatic or allergic attack, may also help them to cope better.

Coping with a chronically sick child

One very important way for some families to cope with chronic and long-term illness in a child is to try to make life as normal as possible. Some people outside the family may see this as a denial of the true situation and therefore as not advisable. The family may well have accepted the meaning of the diagnosis and the poor prognosis but have come to a positive decision to try to make the best of life. One mother told me that her disabled child would only have problems as a result of other people's actions. She was determined that her child could be treated as normal and not create unnecessary difficulties. She was also keen to maintain normal family activities for the siblings, so the disabled child was included whenever possible in their social life. Ray and Ritchie (1993) found that some health professionals do not help parents when they encourage this normalisation. It may be easier, and seem kinder, for professionals to collude with parents' denial of the real problems than to challenge their chosen way of managing. However, some confusion may arise if individual professionals appear to give differing messages regarding the reality of the situation. Each individual family has to make their own judgement about the balance between trying to have a normal life and understanding the reality of the situation with appropriate guidance and support.

Respite care, whether it be for a few hours a week to allow the mother to go shopping or to spend time with other children, an evening out for a treat, or the chance of a week away, may be a greatly valued help to a family. It can break up the sometimes tedious responsibility of constant caring, offering time to renew physical and emotional energies and to look afresh at their ways of coping day to day.

THE ROLE OF HEALTH PROFESSIONALS

The role of health professionals must be to support the family with whatever help is needed and to strengthen the family's own ways of coping with a situation. Purssell (1994) commented that such a large range of skills is needed that it is perhaps not surprising that a positive attitude is not always experienced. Personally, I advocate Rogers' (1961) person-centred approach, which involves demonstrating a 'warm positive regard' for the family members and supporting them in using their own strengths and personal qualities both to cope with their ill child and, at the same time, to maintain a good quality of life for all the family.

It may be helpful to spend time with the parents, reflecting on what has happened in the past and what is happening now, and discussing their current primary concerns, the changes that have taken place and how they feel about these changes. Quite often a family will be unable to appreciate the changes that have occurred, because they have been with the sick child constantly. Whatever means of coping parents found helpful previously may not be appropriate now. Their need for information may change according to how they are feeling or the child's changing condition.

After her research into coping strategies for mothers, Jennings (1992b) concluded: 'it therefore seems necessary for all health professionals involved with mothers of children with life-threatening conditions to organise support that is adequate for that mother's personal needs'. It is clear that, not only mothers, but also the sick child and all other family members, need help to cope with the many and varied difficulties, taking account of the dynamics of their family.

REFERENCES

Berne, E. (1964) *Games People Play*. London: Penguin.
Brown, D. & Pedder, J. (1979) *Introduction to Psychotherapy; an Outline of Psychodynamic Principles and Practice*. London: Tavistock Publications.
Carver, C., Scheier, M. & Weintraub, J. (1989) Assessing coping strategies: a theoretically based approach. *Journal of Personality and Social Psychology*, 56, 267–283.
Chodoff, P., Friedman, S. & Hamburg, D. (1964) Stress, defenses and coping behavior: observations in parents of children with malignant diseases. *American Journal of Psychiatry*, **120**, 743–749.

Eiser, C. (1990) *Chronic Childhood Disease – an Introduction to Psychological Theory and Research.* Cambridge: Cambridge University Press.

Elliot, M. (1981) Parent care. In *Living with Death and Dying*, ed. Kübler-Ross, E. London: Souvenir Press.

Folkman, S. & Lazarus, R.S. (1980) An analysis of coping in a middle aged community sample. *Journal of Health and Social Behaviour*, **21**, 219–239.

Folkman, S. & Lazarus, R. S. (1985). If it changes it must be a process: a study of emotion and coping during three stages of a college examination. *Journal of Personality and Social Psychology*, **48**, 150–170.

Freud, A. (1936). *The Ego and Mechanisms of Defence.* London: Hogarth Press.

Freud, S. (1894) *The Neuro-Psychoses of Defence.* (1) *Standard edition of the complete psychological works of Sigmund Freud*, Vol. 3. London: Hogarth Press and The Institute of Psychoanalysis.

Jacobs, M. (1982) *Still Small Voice.* London: SPCK.

Jennings, P. (1992a) Coping mechanisms. *Paediatric Nursing*, **4(8)**, 13–15.

Jennings, P. (1992b) Coping strategies for mothers. *Paediatric Nursing*, **4 (9)**, 24–26.

Judd, D. (1989) *Give Sorrow Words – Working with a Dying Child.* London: Free Association Books.

Lansky, S. (1974) Childhood leukaemia – the psychiatrist as a member of the oncology team. *American Journal of Child Psychiatry*, **13**, 499–508.

Lazarus, R. (1966) *Psychological Stress and the Coping Process.* New York: McGraw-Hill.

Lazarus, R. (1974) Psychological stress and coping in adaptation and illness. *International Journal of Psychology in Medicine*, **4**, 321–323.

Montagne, L. & Pawlak, R. (1990) Stress and coping of parents of children in a pediatric intensive unit. *Heart and Lung*, **19**, 416–421.

Nelson-Jones, R. (1982) *The Theory and Practice of Counselling Psychology.* London: Cassell.

Noble-Jamieson, G., Cook, P., Parkinson, G. & Barnes, N. (1996) Coping strategies in parents of children receiving liver transplants. *Clinical Child Psychology and Psychiatry*, **1(4)**, 563–573.

Purssell, E. (1994) The process of normalisation in children with chronic illness. *Paediatric Nursing*, **6**, 26–28.

Ray, L. & Ritchie, J. (1993) Caring for chronically ill children at home: factors that influence parents' coping. *Journal of Pediatric Nursing*, **8**, 217–225.

Rogers, C. (1961) *On Becoming a Person.* London: Constable.

Rycroft, C. (1968) *A Critical Dictionary of Psychoanalysis.* London: Penguin.

Schepp, K. (1991). Factors influencing the coping effort of mothers of hospitalized children. *Nursing Research*, **40**, 42–6.

Spufford, M. (1989) *Celebration.* London: Fount Paperbacks.

Turk, J. (1964) Impact of cystic fibrosis on family functioning. *Paediatrics*, **34**, 67–71.

3 Anger

INTRODUCTION

It is essential that nurses, doctors and other carers are aware of the importance of recognising anger, because they are often at the receiving end of much unwanted anger – usually from patients and their families. It is common to be angry with the person who delivers unwelcome or unexpected news, as if that person were responsible for the hurt it has caused. This chapter considers some of the issues around anger in relation to sick children, their families and those caring for them.

UNDERSTANDING ANGER

Over 100 years ago Darwin (1872) recognised anger as one of six basic emotions – happiness, sadness, anger, fear, disgust and surprise. Anger has been described as a primary emotion (Rycroft, 1968), provoked typically by frustration. Although it is often confused with hate, which is a lasting sentiment, anger is in fact a short-lasting emotion easily directed towards those we love. Anger is a feeling of extreme displeasure, hostility, indignation or exasperation towards someone or something (Stewart, 1997).

Kushner (1981) wrote: 'Sometimes, if we cannot find another person to dump our anger on, we turn it on ourselves ... depression is anger turned inward instead of being discharged outward.' He continued by stressing the value of being angry at the situation, rather than ourselves, because the latter makes us depressed:

Being angry at the situation, recognising it as something totally undeserved, shouting about it, denouncing it, crying over it, permits us to discharge the anger which is part of being hurt, without making it harder for us to be helped.

Jacobs (1986) stated that: 'people who fear their anger tend to bottle it up, but have to let go of it every now and again. Controlling anger by suppressing it seldom works for long.' Like the bucket that is getting too full, it will sooner or later overflow.

Anger is frequently off-loaded on to the hospital staff simply because they are there; they are not involved with the family dynamics, so they offer a safe place to dump bad feelings.

It is not unusual for someone going through a difficult time of mixed emotions to split 'good' and 'bad' feelings. The good feelings are directed towards an idealised person and the 'bad' feelings are directed towards someone else, a 'bad' person, possibly even the self (see Case Study 3.1). Jacobs (1986) stated that:

Just as the degree of idealisation is proportionate to the strength of rage, unconsciously felt but repressed, or split off to another person (an equal but opposite force), so rage is proportionate to the degree of need and its consequent frustration.

CASE STUDY 3.1   *Splitting*

For one distressed father, the risk of sharing his anger with the nurses looking after his child, with whom he had built up a good relationship, was very frightening. One morning he told me how angry he had felt towards an agency night nurse looking after his child. He had thought she was not a good nurse because she performed certain tasks differently from the usual nurses, and he had become so annoyed that he had had to go for a walk after midnight. I knew that the nurse had been perfectly capable and was not at fault, but she was an unfamiliar face to the father and therefore a safe target for his increasing anger. His anger was not directed at her in any case; he was angry that his child was seriously ill and suffering and would probably die. It was interesting that he made a particular point of telling me the next morning, dumping his bad feelings about himself onto me!

FRUSTRATION

Frustration is a common cause of anger for the parents of a sick child, who often experience a sense of helplessness when they can do nothing to change the situation. They may become envious of families who appear to have smooth, happy lives, since their own careers and leisure activities will have been interrupted as they struggle to keep the home running and to cope with the sick child.

There is frustration with 'the system', which at times appears to lack efficient communication and cooperation, which makes them wait and which does not give them the answers they seek. It is not uncommon for parents in hospital to complain about the cleaning or the food – subjects they understand – when the really big issues of the child's medical condition and prognosis may be uncertain. The frustration leads them to pin their anger on something tangible – complaining to somebody is at least doing something.

Jacobs (1986), writing to help counsellors understand their clients' frustrations, suggested they should: 'rehearse with such clients ways of expressing their frustration, which include their concern and respect for the other, yet which still convey their own point of view'.

FEAR OF ANGER

There can be great fear of one's own anger, a threatening fear of it getting out of control and erupting at an inappropriate time. This is a very real fear, as illustrated by the numbers of angry parents who damage themselves or verbally or physically abuse staff.

It is possible that this fear of anger is, in fact, a fear of provoking criticism for showing such powerful emotions. Family members may feel that by behaving in a way that is open to criticism from those caring for the sick child, they may be jeopardising the child's care. I have seen parents take avoiding action such as going jogging around the hospital grounds, hitting a pillow and taking a shower (see Case Study 3.2).

CASE STUDY 3.2 Taking action to avoid anger

One mother went up and down in the hospital lift for half an hour – as she put it, 'to calm me down'. She felt safe with strangers in the lift, and just kept going up and down until she felt able to return. Later that evening she commented how she remembered, when she was a child, being sent to her bedroom until she was calm enough to return.

FINDING SOMEONE TO BLAME

When a child is admitted to hospital, seriously ill with meningitis for example, it is common for parents to be angry with their GP thinking that the child had a cold and not sending him to hospital earlier. The fact that there were no signs of meningism before now seems irrelevant to them – they need someone or something to blame for what has happened.

A couple with a child known to have an inherited condition will be offered genetic counselling and tests to investigate the risks of any future babies being affected. This process may lead to the discovery of a 'faulty' gene in one partner, which would then lead to one parent blaming the other for the condition.

In the case of a child who has been knocked down by a car, the parents may be angry with the car driver or with the friend who encouraged their child to run across the road. They are likely to be angry that it was their child, and not someone else's, who was hit and that it happened when they were not present. Their anger may be suppressed by guilt: 'I should have been with her; it would not have happened if I had taken her to school myself.'

Sometimes, anger is simply directed blindly or onwards, at 'everyone'. When I commented to a mother that I thought she had been rather quiet the previous day, she smiled and said she had felt very angry, angry with everyone, and did not want to talk to any of us. The results of investigations had shown that her small son had a malignant tumour and she was understandably angry that this could happen.

It must also be acknowledged that a parent may be angry with the child for having the illness, for causing the accident, or for not wearing the cycle helmet, and this anger may provoke considerable guilt.

ANGER WITH GOD

Anger is often aimed at God, for having allowed this terrible thing to happen; some parents will not speak to the hospital chaplain, who they may consider as representing Him. One father was so distressed that he joked about his son's accident, wondering why God had chosen to have his day off on that particular day. Kushner (1981) echoed the thoughts of many parents who have suffered the serious illness or death of their child: 'I have to believe in God ... so that I have someone to blame, someone to curse and shout at, when I think what I have gone through.'

ANGER AND LOSS

Anger is an important part of the grieving process, whatever the loss or unwelcome change in circumstances. Kübler-Ross (1969), while describing the stages in mourning, observed that anger often emerges when earlier denial and numbness fades. This may be followed by a phase of bargaining and a period of depression, before the emergence of some form of acceptance of the loss.

When parents are at different stages in the grieving process at the same time, it can put an extra strain on the relationship, as one may not understand how the other feels, especially if one of them is angry.

CHILDREN'S ANGER

Children react angrily when they feel misunderstood. A boy recently bereaved of a sibling was confused because he did not know why he felt the way he did. He was angry when relatives told him 'to be a big boy' and when a teacher said he should be 'over it by now'. He did not know what to do and the easiest solution for him at the time was to say nothing and walk away. This did not help him.

Children do not like being left out of family discussions on important topics, especially when it affects them. Many children talk, sometimes years later, of their anger at not being considered important enough to be told the truth about the illness or death of a close family member or friend.

The paediatric patient is likely to be angry about a long-term condition, especially if it means having a different way of life from his peers. It is not surprising, therefore, that a large number of teenagers will rebel against having to take regular drugs, inhalers, insulin injections or special diets. They want to be like everyone else, not in a wheelchair, not having special feeds pumped down a gastrostomy tube overnight, and not having to be absent from school for hospital visits or physiotherapy; they want to be having fun – going to discos, playing sport and wearing clothes like their friends. Older children and adolescents, struggling with the inner turmoil of coping with a distorted body image and sense of worthlessness, also have to deal with the reactions of society, which can be insensitive and rejecting (Judd, 1989).

Bowlby (1973) considered the aggressive behaviour of children who have experienced a separation to be directed towards a parent or parent substitute and to be an expression of the way they have been treated: 'Sometimes it is the anger of hope; sometimes the anger of despair'. He described the hostile play of children who were separated from parents; they frequently attacked dolls they had previously identified as mother or father dolls.

Sick children frequently address their anger to the parent who is there at the time. Many parents, particularly mothers, have been found in tears after a sick child in hospital has made some attack, such as screaming, swearing, biting or hitting. For parents struggling with their own emotions and fears, it is often 'the last straw' when their child shouts 'I hate you!' Lansdown (1996) suggested that the child is expressing a hatred of the fact that the all-powerful parent could not prevent the illness and now cannot provide a cure.

Anger is often suppressed, perhaps unconsciously, by hospital staff and parents in their attempts to make the child's environment as jolly as possible (Judd, 1989). Hospital play specialists, psychologists and play therapists are among those who enable children to act out their feelings and express anger by communicating it through play and drawings. It is commonly said (Winnicott, 1964) that children work off hate and aggression in play, as if aggression were some bad substance inside that could be got rid of. It is, however, important that a child is able to express hate or aggressive urges in a familiar environment, without those feelings being reflected by that environment.

SIBLING ANGER

I spent some time with the older siblings of one particular child who died after being hit by a car. One of them was certainly angry – 'because it happened, because it happened to my sister, to our family'. We talked about how it felt to be angry, and what things helped. One sibling found that it helped to talk to a school friend whose father had died recently. The friend said he punched an old teddy bear when he felt angry. At this point, the children burst out laughing and laughed a lot about this poor old battered bear being punched. One of them said it ached to laugh, because they had not laughed since their sister died. But it was good to laugh – 'you either laugh or cry,' one said. I sensed that this laughing was a great release. We talked about safe ways of dealing with anger, such as kicking a football, or hitting a punch-ball or pillow, and we agreed that kicking the cat or throwing plates was not appropriate.

Bereaved siblings' groups sometimes carry out activities that enable the children to express their anger. The children make large drawings as targets for their angry feelings. At first they may not think of much to include on their drawings, but as we talk with them individually, they begin to remember in greater detail. The child who draws an enormous medicine bottle, bigger than any of the figures, and with the doses and times clearly labelled, probably feels that his family life has been dominated by medicines. There are often strong feelings towards hospitals and doctors who could not make a brother or sisters better. Drips and needles also often provoke unpleasant memories of a sibling's treatment and thus become targets for anger.

Sometimes, anger may be quite strongly directed towards the sibling who is sick or injured – for causing all this fuss, for taking the mother's attention, for interfering with normal life and for getting extra treats and gifts.

MANAGING OTHER PEOPLE'S ANGER

When anger is directed inappropriately at a person, it stirs anger and resentment in that person. In our own families and with friends, we are likely to argue with the angry person or perhaps discuss the cause of their anger, but in our professional situation, we need to be prepared to absorb misdirected anger. We are the convenient hooks on which parents and others hang their anger; it is our job to accept it and defuse it. Sometimes all we can do is acknowledge it calmly. Above all, we must listen (Stewart, 1997).

Working with angry people is tiring and sometimes tests the limits of one's patience; it is therefore important to acknowledge one's own feelings. Those of us who are unable to express our angry feelings openly may find it helpful to write them down on paper, perhaps just as single words in a 'brainstorming' way. The piece of paper can then either be kept, adding more words or crossing words out as appropriate, or it may be therapeutic to tear it into little pieces and throw them away.

Aggressive behaviour resulting from anger is usually acute and does not last long. In health care settings such as hospitals or clinics, it would be sensible to assess the risks to the aggressor and others and to identify the cause of the anger. Occasionally it may be necessary to have help from security personnel and means of restraint.

CONCLUSION

Anger is not always recognised, acknowledged or understood by those needing support and those who are providing it. Sick children and their families and carers may have many reasons to be angry at something or someone, and their responses may be inappropriate or misdirected. By understanding the origin and focus of the anger, the person providing support is more likely to remain calm. This then enables the troubled person to consider the problems more effectively, perhaps with the support of someone who does not appear vulnerable to the angry thoughts and feelings.

REFERENCES

Bowlby, J. (1973) *Attachment and Loss: volume two. Separation: Anxiety and Anger.* Harmondsworth: Penguin.

Darwin, C. (1872) *The Expression of the Emotions in Man and Animals.* London: John Murray.

Kübler-Ross, E. (1969) *On Death and Dying.* London: Tavistock/Routledge.

Kushner, H.S. (1981) *When Bad Things Happen to Good People.* London: Pan Books.

Jacobs, M. (1986). *The Presenting Past – an Introduction to Practical Psychodynamic Counselling.* London: Harper and Row.

Judd, D. (1989). *Give Sorrow Words: Working with a Dying Child.* London: Free Association Books.

Lansdown, R. (1996) *Children in Hospital – a Guide for Family and Carers.* Oxford: Oxford University Press.

Rycroft, C. (1968) *A Critical Dictionary of Psychoanalysis.* London: Penguin.

Stewart, W. (1997) *An A–Z of Counselling Theory and Practice.* Cheltenham: Stanley Thornes.

Winnicott, D. (1964) *The Child, the Family and the Outside World.* London: Penguin.

FURTHER READING

Farrell, G. & Gray, C. (1992) *Aggression, a Nurses' Guide to Therapeutic Management.* London: Scutari.

Fear and anxiety

4

> *The only thing we have to fear is fear itself*
> (Franklin D. Roosevelt)

INTRODUCTION

Fear is one of the most powerful emotions experienced by families of a very sick child, and it is expressed in many different forms. We should take the time to understand a little of what they might be feeling. It is not easy for parents to say how frightened they really are, but it is important to realise the value of allowing them to acknowledge this. They may need permission and encouragement to be honest with themselves, especially in front of strangers who also have some responsibility for their child.

THE IMPORTANCE OF TRUST AND HONESTY

Winnicott (1986), addressing a meeting of doctors and nurses in 1970, suggested:

> ...there is a great deal of potential feedback from psychiatric to general medicine. Psychoanalysis is not just a matter of interpreting the repressed unconscious; it is rather the provision of a professional setting for trust, in which such work can take place.

I believe, because parents have told me so, that trust is of the utmost importance for a good relationship between the family and the professionals caring for their child. Trust will not develop without honesty, and unless we can be trusted to be honest, families may fear that we are hiding the truth.

Winnicott (1986) continued:

> We are dead honest, truthful, saying we do not know when we do not know. An ill person cannot stand our fear of the truth. If we fear the truth, let us take up another profession. By being reliable persons professionally, we protect our patients from the unpredictable. Behind unpredictability lies mental confusion, and behind that there can be

found chaos in terms of somatic functioning, i.e. unthinkable anxiety that is physical.

These wise words ring true for all of us working with families, but particularly in areas of uncertainty, with perhaps frequent changes in a child's condition and treatment. Accident service departments and intensive care units hold many fears for patients and families, but so do visits to the outpatients department and the sometimes unbearable periods spent waiting for results of scans and other diagnostic tests.

PARENTAL FEARS

Fear of the unknown

Fear of the unknown is particularly frightening – so much is uncertain, so much is unpredictable. The parents of a child with severe head injuries are usually desperate to know if the child will survive, and if so, whether there will be any brain damage. If there is any brain damage, then what will that mean – help with walking or feeding? It is too frightening to consider any possibilities worse than that; this is the fear of the nightmare becoming a reality. Somehow, the distressed person has to be supported through the uncertainty with trust and honesty. It is helpful for parents to share their frustrations and fears, to allow someone else to help them to cope with their fears and anxiety. They need help to recognise that hospital staff may not have the answers to their many questions, that there is no crystal ball to foretell the future, nor a magic wand to make everything better. This brings us back to the fear of an uncertain future; if the distant future is too frightening, then parents should be encouraged to concentrate on the very near future – to think about today, not tomorrow or next week or next month.

Fear of a strange environment

For a lay person with no previous experiences on which to draw, a sudden visit to a child needing intensive care or recovering on a ward after an operation can provoke tremendous anxiety. In addition to the apprehension of what they might see, or be expected to do, the room itself, with all its equipment, such as drips, pumps and machines can be frightening (see Case Study 4.1). Considerable help can be offered to reduce these fears, by, for example, talking about the environment and equipment before they go in, and particularly about the child's appearance. Instant photographs can be useful in this situation.

CASE STUDY 4.1   *Fear of the hospital environment*

Margaret's worst fears had come true – she was in hospital with her 4-year-old daughter and it was too much to bear. The child was not seriously ill and only needed to be in hospital for a few days. The biggest difficulty for Margaret was the hospital environment – she was scared and suspicious of everything. She asked about any 'nasty germs' that could come in through the door, on a trolley or on nurses' shoes. 'What was that noise? What was that smell?' Questions all the time. Considerable patience was needed to answer her, and gradually the trust developed.

Fear of losing a child

Most parents of sick children have underlying fears of losing them, although they may not be able to acknowledge these fears. It can be helpful for them to express how they feel and to be reassured by staff, relatives and friends who understand. Case Studies 4.2–4.4 present typical examples of parents' fears.

CASE STUDY 4.2   *Reassurance does not always help fear of loss*

The mother of a child in status asthmaticus was shaking too rigorously to hold a cup of tea when her child needed ventilator assistance for her breathing. All she could whisper was: 'She is my daughter and I love her so much.' She was so frightened that, despite careful explanation of all the equipment and procedures and lengthy attempts to reassure her that the child's airway and breathing were now secure, her overriding concern was of losing her daughter.

CASE STUDY 4.3   *Fear of loss and spoiling*

The parents of a child with a congenital liver disease told how they were so frightened of losing him, as he was such a sick baby, that they had spoiled him. Now, as a result, there would be problems in store when he went home well after a successful liver transplant, instead of being able to enjoy an improved quality of life with the family.

CASE STUDY 4.4   *Rationalising earlier fears*

When given time to talk about her child who had just died from a sudden severe illness, a mother explained that she had always thought she would lose him. He seemed to be accident-prone and had survived a few accidents in the past. Even though he was 10 years old, she kept him beside her as much as possible. He even slept in her bed, as she wanted him close to her – she feared she would not have him long.

Fear of the future

This falls into two categories. First, parents may fear that there will be no future for them and their child at all, i.e. that the child may die. If that possibility is removed, parents may then begin to worry about the kind of future to expect. What will it be like – will the child get better or will there be brain damage? And if so, how severe is it likely to be?

Parents of children with special needs often worry about what will happen to the child when they, his parents and main carers, die. Who, they wonder, will care for him when they are not able to?

Fear of not coping

Parents sometimes fear that they will be unable to cope with the situation, and worry about the humiliation that such an inability will cause (see Case Study 4.5).

CASE STUDY 4.5   Fear of not coping

A very distressed mother told me: 'I do so want to cope. I do try, I can't bear pathetic women. I don't want to not cope. What will my husband think of me? He needs me to cope.' She continued to express quite justifiable feelings about how awful it had been since her severely handicapped baby had been born. She carried enormous guilt for having him, and for being upset when she had two other beautiful children and a high standard of living. During a long tearful session, she told me a great deal about herself and we were able to focus on her many strengths and previously successful coping abilities. I felt that, by the end of an hour, she was less threatened by her fear of the future and how she would cope, as she became more positive about herself. She even talked about how she would like to be able to help other mothers in a local support group.

CHILDREN'S FEARS

Children have their fears too, and those who work with children learn to recognise behaviour resulting from fear (see Case Study 4.6). Preparing children for procedures and new experiences is essential to help allay their fear of the unknown. Hospital play specialists encourage children to look at pictures, and use toys and games to familiarise them with particular equipment and procedures. Specially adapted dolls and teddy bears are used to explain parts of the body that will have an operation scar and where tubes and drips may be sited. The fear seems to fade when a friendly teddy bear is the patient. Many children have real fears of needles and it is well worth spending time with a play specialist or nurse who will allow the children to handle the syringes and needles and 'take blood' from the teddy. Techniques

CASE STUDY 4.6   Identifying children's fears

Following a major abdominal operation, an 8-year-old boy was showing signs of distress. His pain was well controlled, and after further questioning it was ascertained that the drainage tubes were the cause of the problem. He had been watching the blood-stained serous fluid passing down the tube and was afraid that his body was 'melting' and disappearing into the bag at the side of his bed.

can be learned and practised which give the child some control and ways of managing what can be a traumatic event.

Brothers and sisters of a sick child may develop strong fears that they will suffer the same illness, possibly when they reach the same age: 'Will I get leukaemia when I am eight?' It is important, when telling a child about the sibling's illness, to explain that it does not mean they will get it too, and that they are not responsible for what has happened.

Fear caused by pain

Pain can be very frightening for children, especially if it is sudden, such as when waking up after an operation and realising that something is different. They will not have experienced this before and will not know what it means. Children who need their tonsils taken out may be used to having sore or swollen throats, but should be prepared for a different kind of pain when, for example, they first start to drink after the operation. Adequate analgesia should prevent the feeling of panic on experiencing the pain.

Fear of separation and dying

The sick child may develop a fear of dying and being separated from parents and siblings. The parents themselves may find this too frightening to think about and so may not allow the child any opportunity to talk about the feelings that have developed. It is known that adults try to protect children, and themselves, by pretending that all will be well, leading to mutual pretence and protection between the child and adults (Bluebond-Langner, 1978; Muller, Harris and Wattley, 1986; Judd, 1989; While, 1989; Strang, 1989; Lansdown, 1996). Lansdown (1996) reminds us that as children near their teens, there may be more fear and more anger.

If dying is a serious possibility, it is helpful for the parents to have some warning of it: a well-timed explanation of what, how and when it might happen. The fears must be acknowledged;

they are real. Many young parents have not experienced a death in the family; they do not know what to expect and it is likely that they have not seen a dead body before – it is especially frightening to think of their child dying. (It is interesting that many parents who have watched their child die then say that they are now not afraid of dying themselves.) The child who has been in hospital may develop a fear of being left there, and become clingy. After discharge home, it is common for young children to be afraid of going to bed alone, and to be afraid of being left with other people or at nursery school.

Children do not like being left out of important discussions, especially when it concerns them or their family, so it is important that they have good explanations of what is happening. If children are not given answers to their questions or the appropriate information, they will make it up. These imagined situations can be far more frightening than the truth.

FEARS AMONGST THE STAFF

Those who work with children frequently have anxious feelings resulting from their responsibility for the child. Did I answer that question correctly? Have I administered the correct dosage? Have I done the best for the family? Fears of making a mistake are particularly high in intensive care and high-dependency areas, and it is often in these areas that nurses not experienced in children's care feel out of their depth. Continuing support is valuable, in the form of clinical supervision and staff counselling, either individually or within a group.

ANXIETY

Anxiety and fear are closely related emotions that occur frequently and are a normal response to stressful life events. When we are anxious about something, we often say we are worried and we think about the problem until it is resolved. Fear is heightened anxiety, usually as a result of danger or a threat to life or well-being. According to Stewart (1997), anxiety is 'a distressing feeling of uneasiness, apprehension or dread. The fear may be rational, based on an actual event, or irrational, based on an anticipated event which may or may not take place.' Thus, in the case of parents, their anxiety may stem either from their knowledge or previous experience of a situation or from their fears and fantasies of a situation or event that is new to them.

Oliver (1993) discussed the humanistic approach to anxiety and defence of Rogers (1951), who considered that psychological tension arises when individuals cannot assimilate their experiences into their current self-structure. Anxiety was seen by Kelly (1955) as the result of the individual having 'a construction system' that fails him because certain experiences lie outside the scope of existing constructs, therefore making future events difficult to anticipate.

For the families of sick children then, anxiety is to be expected; it is understandable that parents should be worried about their children. Individual family members might benefit from help in acknowledging and managing their own personal anxiety. For this reason, it is important for health professionals to appreciate the parents' feelings and understand the reactions rather than label them as difficult or neurotic.

Symptoms of anxiety

Body reactions often accompany anxiety, and some of these are obvious to the observer. Common symptoms are listed in Box 4.1. These physical symptoms may increase the anxiety if the person thinks they are related to a serious condition, and so much reassurance may be needed; a medical examination to exclude any illness may also be necessary. If there is no underlying medical condition, anxiety usually falls into definite states:

- free floating anxiety, when the person is aware of being overwhelmed by it
- specific anxiety focused on a particular cause, e.g. a child's operation, loss of a job
- a phobia
- panic disorder
- post-traumatic stress disorder.

Box 4.1   Common symptoms of anxiety

- Tension of body, limbs or facial muscles
- Tightness in the chest
- Distress, e.g. crying
- Irritability and impatience
- Loss of concentration; the person is easily distracted
- Easily tired
- Difficulty in sleeping
- Muscle pains
- Inability to relax
- Sweating, pallor or flushing

- Hyperventilation
- Fainting and dizziness
- Nausea, indigestion, difficulty swallowing
- Bowel disturbances, urgency
- Frequency in passing urine
- Palpitations

Phobias

A phobic is someone who shows signs of intense anxiety and panic in specific situations. Generally they will:

- become anxious and fearful out of all reasonable proportion
- not be able to give or discuss explanations and reasons for their anxiety
- not be able to control the panic voluntarily
- avoid the feared object or situation.

It is not easy for, say, a mother to come to hospital with her child if she has a phobia of hospitals. She may not be able to watch the child have an injection or blood test if she cannot stand the sight of needles, or go up several floors in a lift if she cannot bear to be shut in a confined space. Parents may need to be understood and well supported by staff so that they are not seen to let the child down. They might benefit from talking through their fears and looking at ways of overcoming the phobia, such as a gradual reintroduction to a task or situation they fear with someone they trust alongside them. A psychologist or counsellor may help with behavioural or desensitisation skills.

Some children have real fears of needles, while others, who have a long-term illness or need frequent blood tests, may develop needle phobia, especially if there have been repeated attempts at gaining access to a vein or the child has been hurt. Hospital play specialists use techniques to help children overcome this fear by playing with dolls and teddy bears and real syringes and needles. The children play the role of the nurse or doctor, handling the syringes and needles and giving the teddy a blood test or injection. They can also speak the part of teddy, thus expressing their own fears through a friendly bear. Once the child can cope with the sight of the needles and is familiar with how they are used, it becomes easier to plan with the child the best way of managing the actual blood test, allowing her to have some control over the procedure.

Panic

A sudden onset of great anxiety and fear leads to panic when the anxiety becomes intolerable. Anticipation of the dreaded sight or event alone may bring on panic attacks (see Case Study 4.7).

CASE STUDY 4.7   Panic attacks

Jane's little daughter was critically ill in the children's intensive unit. Her husband was not able to stay overnight with her because he went home to be with their older child. When she woke up in the mornings, she could not bring herself to ring the unit to ask how her daughter was, as she was always afraid of hearing bad news. Instead, she would get dressed quickly and rush to the unit. By the time she reached the doors of the corridor outside, she would be shaking and finding it hard to walk in the right direction. When she reached the door of the unit, she would freeze and start hyperventilating; there was no way she could push the door open herself. She waited until someone else opened the door to go in or out so she could see in first. Jane talked about her difficulty and said she felt silly but was extremely afraid that her child's condition may have deteriorated and was too scared to go in and find out. She would feel guilty that she had left her, and in her panic would think: 'What if she had died and I didn't know?'

The importance of talking about fears and feelings

Freud (1894) first thought that defence caused anxiety, but he later changed his mind, thinking that defence was in fact provoked by anxiety:

Anxiety is the commonest form of distress from which we can suffer ... a situation which, prolonged, produces disturbances of physiology and of mental equilibrium which can become intolerably destructive.

Freud believed that the sources of anxiety, together with the feelings aroused by them, could be repressed and that the entire constellation of feelings and experience could be banished from consciousness and pre-consciousness into the unconscious area of the mind. It was their partial, distorted or disguised re-emergence under pressure which produced the symptoms of hysteria: 'a conversion from repressed anxiety to overt but quite changed experience of loss or distortion of function' (Stafford-Clark, 1965).

Everyone suffers from anxiety; it is part of our lives from the moment of birth when we experience the anxiety of separation from our mothers or simply the anxiety of not being held securely (Winnicott, 1958). For those of us who work with people going through unexpected and deeply emotional periods causing anxiety, it is important to consider Freud's beliefs that the sources of anxiety and the feelings can be banished from consciousness and reappear later. It would seem beneficial to encourage distressed people to talk about their fears and feelings at the time they are actually experiencing them, to acknowledge the bad feelings and set about dealing with them, rather than denying them and trying to bury them.

OVERCOMING ANXIETY

Not all anxiety is bad. It can increase our awareness of a situation and is a normal emotion at a stressful time. A helper may need to allow the anxious person to stay with the anxiety for a while and to support them in this by helping them to manage it and not be afraid of it. Winnicott (1986) describes this as a complex kind of 'holding' – the professional therapist or nurse steps in to help when the patient is failing to cope.

Most people need to know what is wrong and how it can be put right. This usually means learning something about themselves, in particular:

- What makes them anxious?
- Why does this make them anxious?
- What has gone on before, and how do those events relate to the present situation?

Having an understanding of the meaning and significance of events is necessary before a person can develop her own control and management of the anxiety.

An anxious person does not usually live in isolation and her situation needs to be considered in the context of her family and her environment. Account needs to be taken of:

- family dynamics
- social support available
- the important issues – e.g. who will care for a well child at home; who will pay the bills; how will I cope?
- the aims or goals – for the sick child and for the family as a whole
- changes which could be made.

Severe anxiety or neuroses may need:

- *Medical intervention*
  — examination and, possibly, investigation, for reassurance
  — drugs (anxiolytics, antidepressants, beta-blockers)
- *Psychological treatment*
  — counselling, psychotherapy (individually or in groups)
  — behavioural therapy – taking away the avoidance

— cognitive behavioural therapy – helpful for panic disorder, some phobias, obsessive compulsive disorder
— creative therapy – expressing anxiety through art, music or drama
— family therapy – working with the whole family
* *Social support* – voluntary and self-help groups, home visits, family support.

Help for children

Children may need help with their anxiety, in the same way as do adults, and their behaviour, moods, and changes in sleeping or eating patterns may suggest that help is required.

Young children usually respond well to skilled play therapy, and children of all ages benefit from individual or family therapy at 'child and family consultation clinics'. Judd (1991) explained that: 'child psychotherapists work with a wide range of children suffering from emotional and behavioural difficulties. They help children to understand their fantasies and feelings, so they can better manage their lives.' Lansdown (1996) believes that the reduction of anxiety is a major function of play in hospital, and that it can be a safety valve for feelings and an outlet for tensions and conflicts. He emphasised the great importance of play guided by a play specialist.

A study by Eiser (1990) of the research evaluating the benefit of preparing children for hospital and procedures indicated that the parental role in shaping the child's response is clearly critical. Eiser suggested that if parents can play a major role in reducing their child's anxiety about procedures, it could be that preparation of parents is the key to the most successful preparation of children.

Identifying the stressors

If the stress factors can be identified and some preparation work carried out before the anticipated event, this usually goes some way towards reducing the anxiety surrounding the event. For some, this means finding out as much information as possible in order to be able to feel in control.

Relaxation

Exercises to relax mind and body can be very helpful for parents, as well as meditation, listening to music and guided imagery. Regular, sensible eating, sufficient sleep and a positive attitude all help in controlling anxiety. Children also benefit from relaxation, which is helped by stroking, rocking, massage, music, guided imagery and listening to stories.

CONCLUSION

Bowlby (1973) studied Freud's theories of anxiety and concluded that there is probably no single key to an understanding of anxiety, as fear and anxiety are aroused in many different situations. It is clear, however, that the particular form of anxiety arising from separation and loss is not only common, but also leads to great and widespread suffering.

Trying to lower the levels of fear and anxiety by understanding their sources is beneficial to both helpers and those being helped. It may take extra time and effort, but it is worth it for the sake of sick children and their families, all of whom are likely to suffer from, or be exposed to, these potentially debilitating emotions.

REFERENCES

Bowlby, J. (1973) *Attachment and Loss: volume two. Separation: Anxiety and Anger.* Harmondsworth: Penguin.

Bluebond-Langner, M. (1978) *The Private Worlds of Dying Children.* Princeton: Princeton University Press.

Eiser, C. (1990) *Chronic Childhood Disease.* Cambridge: Cambridge University Press.

Freud, S. (1894) *The Neuro-Psychoses of Defence.* (1) standard edition of the complete psychological works of Sigmund Freud, vol. 3. London: Hogarth Press and The Institute of Psychoanalysis.

Judd, D. (1989) *Give Sorrow Words – Working with a Dying Child.* London: Free Association Press.

Judd, D. (1991) Rooting for the source of anxiety – child psychotherapy at work. *Professional Nurse,* **6(5),** 252–256.

Kelly, G. (1955) *The Psychology of Personal Constructs,* vol. 1. New York: Norton.

Lansdown, R. (1996) *Children in Hospital.* Oxford: Oxford University Press.

Muller, D. J., Harris, P. J. & Wattley, L. (1986) *Nursing Children: Psychology, Research and Practice.* London: Harper and Row.

Oliver, R. W. (1993) *Psychology and Health Care.* London: Baillière Tindall.

Rogers, C. R. (1951) *Client-centred Therapy, its Current Practices, Implications and Theory.* Boston: Houston.

Stafford-Clark, D. (1965) *What Freud Really Said.* London: Penguin Books.

Stewart, W. (1997) *An A–Z of Counselling Theory and Practice,* 2nd edn. Cheltenham: Stanley Thornes.

Strang, K. (1989) Living through the death of a child. *Nursing Times,* **7,** 39–41.

While, A. E. (1989) The needs of dying children and their families. *Health Visitor,* **62,** 176–178.

Winnicott, D. W. (1958) Anxiety associated with insecurity. In *Collected Papers,* ed. Winnicott, D. W. London: Tavistock.

Winnicott, D. W. (1986) *Home is Where We Start From.* London: Penguin.

5 Guilt and responsibility

INTRODUCTION

The feelings of guilt that some parents describe are incredibly powerful. I believe that this is bound up closely with the responsibility of their being parents. There is a primary responsibility for parents to keep their offspring safe and well, and this is true for all animals. This is why I have chosen to discuss guilt and responsibility in the same chapter; it may be more appropriate to put responsibility first, as guilt will be inevitable if responsibility has not been fulfilled. When a child is sick, and especially if a child dies, the parents' sense of loss relates to their feeling of responsibility for that child – simply because they are the child's parents and not necessarily because they could have prevented it in any way.

Professionals working with families will be familiar with parents expressing guilt. They need to understand what the parents are going through if they are to help them move on and not be dragged down by the enormous weight of the guilt.

Children with congenital or lifelong problems

Parents of children born with physical abnormalities or health problems often describe how they 'feel really guilty, we both do, for making a baby like this'. Later, they may even express guilt for having expected to have a perfectly normal child.

The parents may have been offered prenatal screening and may have chosen not to have this done. They may have known that problems were possible, or even likely, but decided to continue with the pregnancy anyway. This decision is likely to have been taken after much consideration of their responsibility both to the unborn child and also to the other members of the family. However, whatever they thought prior to the birth, the likelihood is that now the baby has been born, their appreciation of the situation will be different.

It is often very difficult for parents to accept that they carry genes for inherited conditions, and they may search for other reasons for the child being born with a particular problem. Environmental causes such as contaminated water supplies, air pollution, and power station and factory emissions are frequently blamed, and sometimes stress or diet during pregnancy is felt to be responsible. This denial of the reality of the problem may continue after the child's birth, or even early death, when parents decide to have another baby without waiting for genetic counselling, as if to prove they can have a normal baby and thereby clear themselves of the guilt.

There may be a need to place the blame with someone or something else. If couples are not able to share this, it can divide them when blame is directed at one side of the family. Grandparents may be keen to show that they are not the guilty party declaring: 'There is none of this on our side of the family.'

On this question of guilt, Clarke (1994) wrote:

It is not surprising that parents can feel guilt for the birth, for the life, and then for the death of their child with a genetic disease. Where a family has one affected child, the subsequent birth of a second affected infant can lead to the explicit labelling of the parents as being irresponsible.

(See also Case Study 5.1).

CASE STUDY 5.1   Sisters with cystic fibrosis

Megan has cystic fibrosis and so does her older sister, although she has always enjoyed much better health and quality of life than Megan. During one of Megan's spells in hospital she became rather depressed about her condition and blamed her parents for having her when they already had a child with cystic fibrosis. Their parents felt this blame very deeply and told Megan that they had chosen to have her, even with cystic fibrosis, and would always love her and care for her. They exhausted themselves with the constant care and attention they gave her.

As children grow older, they develop a greater understanding of their condition and its implications. It is not unusual for teenagers to resent the treatment they need to stay well and to protest by not complying. They may feel guilty at a later stage for causing worry to their parents. Feelings of guilt may be quite strong in a child who is dependent on others for help, but they are likely to be mixed with frustration and anger at being different from everyone else.

Children with acute illness

When a child is seriously ill after a short history of being unwell, as is often the situation with meningitis for example, there is tremendous guilt while the parents come to accept the diagnosis. They ask many questions of themselves: 'Why didn't I notice sooner that something was wrong?'; 'Why didn't I call the doctor earlier?', 'If only I hadn't left him with a friend'; 'If only I had listened to my mother – she said he was ill'. The shock of being rushed into hospital with the dreaded word 'meningitis' ringing in your ears is terrifying enough without the self-inflicted torture of the guilt.

Father's guilt

There is a particular kind of guilt that a father sometimes expresses when his child's life is threatened, growing from a regret of having spent time away from the family because of his work. The fact that he has progressed well in his career, maintained a steady job or earned a regular income seems unimportant when he may lose the child whose future he was working so hard to make secure (see Case Study 5.2).

CASE STUDY 5.2   A father's guilt

John was a kind man who worked hard at his business, which failed despite his efforts. He felt extremely guilty when his child became ill, as he had spent so much time working, but without the results he had hoped for. The guilt grew stronger as his feelings of failure as a father added to his failure at work and he became depressed.

It seemed right to talk with John about what was happening now. Even though there had been serious financial problems in the recent past, he had survived and they had survived as a family. He was there in hospital with his family when they needed him at this difficult time; he had not stayed away.

He found it hard not to be able to plan ahead as he usually set his goals and aimed straight for them, but now he could not see the way forward. We talked about aiming for goals he could reach, even if it was only making a cup of coffee or going out to buy a newspaper. We also discussed the fact that he should not be expecting too much of himself as he was still numb from the shock of a poor prognosis for their child. If he set himself tasks he could not achieve, his sense of failure would grow.

There were positive points to appreciate, but he needed to be reminded of them. He had a good, strong relationship with his wife and children, and his own inner strength had enabled him to cope with previous hard times. He found it helpful to be reassured that he was not abnormal or becoming mentally ill, and to have the opportunity to talk about feelings that seemed unbearable. His overwhelming sense of guilt and failure would have prevented him from coping with each day and what it might bring.

Guilt after accidents or injuries

A guilt reaction is usual and understandable in parents of a child who has been burned or scalded at home. Somehow one expects this sort of accident to be totally preventable when every care is taken to protect children: 'It was my fault, ... she will be scarred for life. I can never forgive myself.'

Apart from feeling guilty at having let the child down, there is also guilt in the face of the other parent's possible disapproval, that somehow the job of caring for the child was not done properly. I have heard mothers apologising to the fathers for what has happened. There is an important link here between guilt and shame. The sense of shame comes from feelings of failure, disappointment and 'letting the side down'.

After accidental injuries, we hear many 'if only' comments. People entertain thoughts such as: 'if only mother or father had taken the child to school that day, he would not have rushed across the road and been hit by a car'; if only I had watched him leave on his bicycle, I would have made him wear his helmet'. Other people who were involved feel guilty too, especially where children are concerned.

Children's guilt

Even young children can feel guilt that in some way events are their fault. For example, they may feel guilty because their sibling or a friend has an illness or disability that perhaps they could have prevented (see Case Study 5.3).

CASE STUDY 5.3   *Guilt at perceived inaction*

Melanie was 8 years old and her sister Kate was 5 when they were at a pony club show. Kate was sitting on a friend's pony when something startled it and she fell off. Adults who were there gave Melanie the pony's reins to hold while they helped her sister and fetched their parents. Kate was taken to hospital and needed many months of special care and rehabilitation. It was over a year later that it became clear that Melanie needed special help to work through her feelings that she might have been able to help her sister, but instead had held the pony's reins, as instructed.

Sick children need the important adults in their lives to acknowledge the illness or condition, to help them accept it, but also to let them know that other people whom they know and trust can also accept it. Some children think they are ill because they are naughty, so they need to be told it was not their fault, nor anyone else's. That responsibility could cause a huge burden of unnecessary guilt. Older children may feel guilty at being in hospital and having their parents visit when they should be at work or at home caring for siblings. Sometimes a holiday or special activity cannot take place because a child is sick, which then makes the child feel guilty and responsible for the others missing a treat.

Survivor guilt

Sometimes, brothers or sisters who are well, or who have survived an accident or disaster in which a sibling was hurt, show signs of 'survivor guilt'. These feelings may be expressed as follows: 'It should have been me who got this illness because Mum likes him more than me. He was the favourite'; or 'I should have been hit by the car as he can run faster than I can'.

Bereaved parents may feel especially guilty that they have survived longer than their child. Grandparents often feel this particularly strongly, having outlived their grandchild who was their hope for the future.

On this question of survivor guilt, Wright (1986) stated:

when one dies in a disaster, the other feels in some way responsible. On a rational and intellectual level the person knows he has no power over such incidents, but he punishes himself with the thought that he has.

(See Case Study 5.4.) Survivor guilt is also discussed in Chapter 11 (p. 148).

CASE STUDY 5.4   Survivor guilt

Simon was so overwhelmed with guilt that he could not talk to anyone and definitely did not want to see his brother Mark in hospital after the accident. Simon had crossed the road before Mark, without waiting for him. His brother did not look before crossing the road and was hit by a lorry. Simon felt he should be blamed for the accident as he had not waited for Mark and had called him across the road.

Guilt in bereavement

Kübler-Ross (1969) described a bargaining stage in grieving; part of the bargaining is about making promises, possibly secretly with God. Psychologically, promises may be associated with unspoken guilt. Bereaved parents are particularly guilt-ridden after the death of their child, often blaming themselves for what has happened.

Kander (1990), addressing bereaved parents, suggested that guilt and conscience are opposite in origin. Conscience is developed from a basis of moral teaching, and having made it our own, it becomes an inner responsibility for our choice of actions. Guilt is from an outer source, originating in the judgement of others or in our expectation of external disapproval; as such, we have the choice not to live with it continuously.

Anger and guilt

Anger is more closely associated with guilt than is perhaps generally thought. Stewart (1997) reminds us that guilt may be anger turned inwards and it is therefore helpful to work with the anger. I witnessed one mother, whose child had been knocked down by a car, become extremely angry at all those around her – her husband, other family members and the nursing and medical staff. It was quite inappropriate. I remember her saying, almost as an aside, that she felt guilty for not being with her child when the accident happened. This guilt was perhaps too large a burden for her to carry alone while she was recovering from the shock of the accident.

Often, a person may react in anger, sometimes physically, even violently, and then suffer guilt and embarrassment about it afterwards; the reason for being angry needs to be acknowledged in order to work through it (Wright 1991) (see Case Study 5.5).

CASE STUDY 5.5   *Guilt and anger*

After I had seen a mother talking on the ward telephone in tears, I went to see her by the child's bed. She was desperately upset because her partner had rung to ask how their child was after the operation and had demanded answers to many questions. When she told him she did not know all the answers, he had shouted at her that she should know – 'you have been at the hospital all day'. When we talked about this unexpected outburst, it was clear that he did not like hospitals and had used the excuse that he had important things to do at work that day, even though he could have taken time off. Perhaps he was feeling guilty for not supporting his partner and child, was angry with himself and frustrated at not getting the answers to his questions.

The anger and guilt felt by parents struggling to care for disabled children may need to be expressed at times when life is hard going. It is not surprising that these feelings get discharged when a target presents itself, such as a doctor giving bad news, a delayed operation, help that does not arrive as promised or the paperwork and time spent in making claims for money to which they may be entitled.

RESPONSIBILITY

I began this chapter by acknowledging the close relationship between guilt and responsibility. Unfortunately, not all parents take the responsible role of parenting seriously enough, while others are tormented by the worry of failing in their duty to the child (see Case Study 5.6).

CASE STUDY 5.6   *Guilt and responsibility*

Maria's baby had been born at 26 weeks' gestation as she was suffering from high blood pressure. The baby spent many weeks in the neonatal intensive care unit before she was taken home for the short time before she died. Some months later, Maria told me how she had been on a slimming diet and had lost weight. She knew that she had been overweight when she was pregnant and that was probably why she had high blood pressure, the reason for her baby being born so early. She felt very guilty about this, saying that her weight was in her control; she should have lost weight for her baby's sake. Maria was now taking this responsibility seriously and was determined to be slimmer before she tried to conceive another baby.

This story illustrates Maria's strong feelings of guilt and responsibility. The strict diet may be seen as a kind of punishment she must undergo before becoming deserving of the wonderful 'prize' of another baby.

Most parents would choose to take full responsibility for their children and to make their own decisions about their welfare, education, diet etc. When something happens in life that results in changes from the normal, such as in illness or injury, this responsibility may have to be shared, e.g. with health professionals. The parents will need a lot of new information and advice and may feel that they are not in control of what is happening. Professionals can help to restore a sense of control by providing the information parents require patiently and carefully, all the while checking that it has been understood.

Some decisions are so great and difficult that it is not right to expect anyone to make them alone. Hopefully, parents will be able to make informed decisions and therefore be responsible. One of the most difficult areas must surely be the decision to withdraw treatment for a child. I recall clearly a mother's plea for help when she said to the doctor: 'Please do not ask me to switch off the ventilator. I cannot be responsible for that.' It was a great relief for her when the consultant said it would be his decision, which he would share with her. She talked later of how she could not have lived with the guilt of being responsible for that decision. Without that burden, she was able to concentrate on the important information being explained to her and to make the most of the remaining time with her child, thus preventing even more regret and guilt afterwards.

Children also develop a sense of responsibility, and feel guilty, angry or ashamed when it appears to them that they might have failed to live up to it. Sick children may feel responsible for their own illness, while siblings often display a desire to be 'good' and 'well' as if to make up for the sick child.

Conclusion

Many feelings of guilt can be eased by sharing them or by talking them through with someone experienced in listening. It may be difficult to express the strong feelings of shame and inadequacy often associated with guilt. They need to be acknowledged and explored, in order to allow a sharing of the responsibility. Psychoanalyists distinguish 'normal' guilt (remorse), which would respond to 'confession', from 'pathological' guilt, for which therapy would be more appropriate (Stewart, 1997).

There are some truly unbearable situations when someone really does appear to be at fault, because of what he did or did not do, with disastrous results, e.g. when a child suffers accidental, or non-accidental, injury. The law may punish a speeding or drunken driver, but a parent responsible for a young child who drowns in a garden pond, suffers bad burns from a kitchen cooker or runs in front of a moving car will be punished by the guilt of having failed to prevent it.

It is hard to imagine how one might help a person (a father, say) so full of guilt; but listening to his story, acknowledging his feelings and accepting him in spite of what he has done may help him to feel that he has not been rejected. It may also help to encourage him to take a broader view of the situation, once again sharing some of the responsibility, with comments such as: 'You acted quickly and did your best to help'; 'We all make mistakes at times'. Independent counselling would probably help such a person to work through some difficult issues, and prevent him spoiling the lives of a partner and surviving children as well as his own.

Unfair criticism and comments from other people sometimes creates guilt, particularly if a person is vulnerable, lacking in self-confidence and generally unable to cope with it, as are many parents with a sick child. Discussing and sharing the difficulties with trusted friends and professionals allow a person to take a wider view of a situation and possibly to reach a more rational understanding.

Caring for children is a huge responsibility, whether as a parent or professional, and must be taken seriously. The *Concise Oxford Dictionary* (1990) gives three definitions of 'responsible':

- liable to be called to account to a person or for a thing
- morally accountable for one's actions, capable of rational conduct
- of good credit, position or repute; evidently trustworthy.

These three points emphasise that we are all responsible for someone or something and have a responsibility to ourselves, and to others, to be reputable and trustworthy. When working with a person suffering from guilt, there is an urgent need to help that person balance conscience with responsibility (Stewart, 1997). When we feel that we have not fulfilled our responsibility, the guilt can be overwhelming; hence the significance of the relationship between responsibility and guilt for families of sick children.

REFERENCES

Clarke, A. (1994) Dying from genetic diseases. In *Caring for Dying Children and Their Families*, ed. Hill, L. London: Chapman and Hall.

Kander, J. (1990) *So will I comfort you*. Cape Town: Lux Verbi.

Kübler-Ross, E. (1969) *On Death and Dying*. London: Tavistock/Routledge.

Stewart, W. (1997) *An A – Z of Counselling Theory and Practice*, 2nd edn. Cheltenham: Stanley Thornes.

Wright, B. (1986) *Caring in Crisis – a Handbook of Intervention Skills for Nurses*. Edinburgh: Churchill Livingstone.

Wright, B. (1991) *Sudden Death*. Edinburgh: Churchill Livingstone.

FURTHER READING

Dryden, W. (1994) *Overcoming Guilt*. London: Sheldon.

Depression

The true opposite of depression is not gaiety or absence of pain, but vitality: the freedom to experience spontaneous feelings.
(Alice Miller, 1987).

INTRODUCTION

Parents of sick children may sometimes be described as being depressed, which is perhaps not surprising when we think about the problems that some of them have to bear. It may therefore be helpful to think about some of the ways depression may present in various situations.

UNDERSTANDING DEPRESSION

The word depression generally refers to either an emotional state or a clinical diagnosis (Rycroft, 1968). In the context of an emotion, there does not seem to be a very clear definition, as the word is frequently used to describe a broad range of feelings. However, it usually implies a lowering of spirits and suggests feelings of being 'bogged down', unable to struggle out of a bad patch, or of sadness or disappointment for longer than expected. The diagnosis and treatment of depressive disorders are not of interest in the context of this book, but health professionals working with sick children and their families need to be aware of the temporary periods of depression which may develop following life changes such as illness, loss, bereavement, trauma and childbirth. It is only by being aware that professionals will be able to help family members to understand what they are going through.

In 1917, Freud drew attention to the similarities between bereavement and depression; in both cases the individual may experience sadness, despair, loss of interest in the outside world and an inhibition of activity (Brown and Pedder, 1979). Freud (1917) habitually used the term 'melancholia' for conditions now described as depression. Jacobs (1986) recognised that depression is sometimes caused by anger turned in on oneself, and that 'the inability to be competitive, sometimes manifested as depressed feelings of being unable to succeed, can cause problems'. Both of these comments are relevant when considering families with sick children.

Winnicott (1963) was taught that:

...depression has within itself the germ of recovery. This is the one bright spot in psychopathology, and it links depression with the sense of guilt (a capacity for which is a sign of healthy development) and with the mourning process. Mourning too tends eventually to finish its job.

There is a feeling of hope here, that within depression itself there is the possibility of recovery, like a seed waiting to be nurtured in order to grow and develop. This is encouraging; the depressed person will probably get better, when the time and conditions are right. When mourning has completed its task, the depression fades. The strong link between a sense of guilt and depression is very relevant for parents, who seem to carry huge burdens of guilt when their child is ill.

DEPRESSION AND GRIEVING

Elisabeth Kübler-Ross (1969) has identified depression as one of the five stages in the grieving process, after denial, bargaining and anger. It is often the time when bereaved persons present at the doctor's surgery with psychosomatic symptoms, insomnia, tiredness and generally feeling down. Bereavement counsellors report that their highest numbers of referrals are for those who are stuck in their grieving, around 3 or 4 months after the loss. This temporary depression allows time to work through the painful issues, often with help, before being able to move on to some degree of acceptance, the final stage of grieving.

We should always bear in mind that grieving is a natural response to loss, and when a child is sick, for whatever reason and for however long, there are losses involved (see Ch. 7) It is inevitable that there will be periods of depression or despair.

DEPRESSION AND COPING WITH TRAUMATIC AND STRESSFUL EXPERIENCES

Parents may become depressed during or after an emotionally difficult event or period in their lives, and it would seem that the likelihood of this occurring is related to the way in which they have coped with the event or period itself. A study by Noble-

Jamieson *et al.* (1996) followed the coping strategies of parents whose children received liver transplants. The parents completed the Beck Depression Inventory (Beck and Steer, 1987) after their child's discharge, in which, in response to specific questions, they described their feelings and attitudes about the experience. It emerged that the parents who became depressed had quite different methods of coping from the other parents. The depressed parents showed considerably greater helplessness, despair and pessimism postoperatively, and greater denial, lack of realism, disappointment, anxiety, helplessness and despair after the child's discharge home.

RECOGNISING SIGNS OF DEPRESSION

Sometimes it is not easy to notice whether a person is depressed. A sulking person may either become antisocial or, indeed, display the opposite behaviour, appearing bright and cheerful when feeling low. Humour may be a defence for depression, particularly when it is inappropriate.

It is not uncommon for people to keep smiling through everything, hiding the bad feelings behind a positive appearance. This is often seen in parents of a child with a chronic condition. However difficult it might be caring for the child and managing the home, when a health professional visits, the parents give the impression that everything is under control. It is therefore difficult for the professional to judge whether life is becoming too difficult for them to manage.

There is a considerably high rate of depression amongst parents of sick children, which is not surprising, but it does perhaps indicate that counselling should be available as part of their package of care, both in hospital and in the community. Having someone to talk to, who will listen, can be of great support to parents, who may be feeling quite isolated and alone with their problems and fears.

Parents who have been through a traumatic time in hospital may drop the facade of appearing to be in control of their emotions when they are back in the relative safety of their home. I have heard mothers say they have booked a nervous breakdown for when they get home! It is well worth warning parents that they might feel down when they get home and are able to relax and reflect on just what they have all been through.

Children can become depressed, even at a very young age. Their behaviour may change from being happy and outgoing to being quiet and withdrawn, and they may lose interest in activities and food that they previously enjoyed. They might have deep fears, perhaps about procedures, pain or even the possibility of their own death, and unless opportunities are given to talk about these, they may try to block them out completely, thinking that this is the only safe way for the dreadful thoughts to be banished.

Box 6.1 presents a series of questions a professional might ask in relation to sick children, their families and their carers as a means of assessing their vulnerability to depression.

Box 6.1   Assessment of vulnerability to depression

Mother
- How is she coping?
- Is practical help available?
- Does she share her thoughts and fears?
- Does she support the father and does he or her partner support her?
- Have there been changes in her behaviour or appearance?
- What is her state of health?
- Is postnatal depression a possibility?

Father
- Does he share the care of the child?
- Does he support the child's mother?
- Do the parents talk and share as a couple?
- Does he use work as an excuse to keep away?
- Is he kept informed?

Siblings
- Are they involved and kept informed?
- Are they encouraged to visit?
- Are they given time to discuss their own feelings?

The sick child
- Are the child's needs being met?
- Is age-appropriate, honest information given?
- Does the family discuss matters openly?
- Is the child allowed to talk about the illness?
- Is a play specialist or counsellor available for the child?

Carers and health professionals
- Are they well supported, by colleagues and by managers?
- Are they given appropriate training and study days?
- Can they share thoughts with colleagues?
- Do they have sufficient resources?

POSTNATAL DEPRESSION

It would be helpful for those involved with mothers and babies to have an understanding of postnatal depression. During the period between 3 months and 1 year after childbirth, this disorder may affect many mothers. The signs may not be noticed amid the excitement and disruption of a new baby, but early recognition will be of significant help in preventing long-term problems.

When all is not well, e.g. if the baby has a congenital abnormality or condition, or becomes ill during the first few months, the anxiety can increase the mother's depression. In this case, other relatives are also anxious and the depression may go on for some months without being noticed. A mother with postnatal depression may have considerable difficulty in bonding with the baby, and when there is a problem with the baby's health this could lead to her rejecting the baby.

Hospital nurses may think that this is a community problem, but they should be aware of the symptoms and be able to give help if a mother is in hospital. Practical advice to the mother and lessons in managing the baby's care, as well as caring for herself, should be available. Time for her to talk to someone who knows how to listen shows that she is important too. She needs to understand that it is all right to have time away from the baby when a friend or relative offers to babysit, to have time with her partner, and to allow herself proper mealtimes and sleep. Supportive friends and relatives who help with other children and who visit frequently will help to minimise the mother's isolation from the outside world.

SADNESS AND DESPAIR

'When you are sorrowful, look again into your heart, and you shall see that in truth you are weeping for that which has been your delight.'
(The Prophet: Gilbran, 1926)

We should remind ourselves that sadness and despair are not the same as depression. There is always some sadness when a child is ill, and the sadness is often shared with other parents, giving valuable support. The health professionals also share this sadness; thankfully, it is now acceptable for nurses to share some emotions with the family receiving bad news about their child. On one occasion, a mother said that even the nurse had tears in her eyes, and this seemed to reinforce the devastating fact that the child was not going to recover from the injuries. It supported the harsh reality of the moment, but above all, the nurse was right there with the parents, sharing their sadness; they felt understood and not alone.

Despair may become apparent at some point, the timing of it depending on the condition of the sick child and the coping abilities of the parents. If progress is minimal or slow, they may begin to lose hope, and it is usually hope that keeps one going through such difficult periods of uncertainty. It is the light at the end of a long dark tunnel, but if there are no signs of improvement, then the tunnel can seem very long and very dark. By acknowledging this darkness and trying to accept the dreadful situation, it may be possible to adopt the positive view that things can only get better. There is some reassurance for parents that, despite the situation being so bad, they have survived.

LOSS OF INTEREST

A mother who had been living in the hospital since her child became ill said: 'I've been stuck in here for 4 weeks now', and as such, was acknowledging her own feeling of despair. For a parent who is 'stuck' in hospital, tied up in the world surrounding a sick child, it is not unusual to lose interest in the world outside. If they are a long distance from home, visits from friends and family may be infrequent, and the main contacts may be through telephone calls. I have heard such mothers make comments like: 'I don't care what the house looks like'; 'I can't remember what is in the freezer, they will just have to manage'. They are rarely interested in reading a newspaper; if they do, they often say it is full of depressing stories. They may not even notice the weather outside and may not consider going for a short walk for a change of environment.

This loss of interest often extends to their personal activities: they may not bother to wash their hair or iron their clothes. They may say things like: 'I am too lazy to go for a proper meal, so I just eat snacks.' Given time to reflect on this, parents would probably recognise that they need proper food to preserve their strength in order to help their child. The health professional can help them to do this.

SUPPORTIVE COUNSELLING

Depression in these circumstances is usually temporary, lifting as the child becomes well again. The counselling role is, for the greater part, a holding and supportive one, acknowledging how a parent feels now, no matter how bad; they may even be suicidal. Parents must feel safe about sharing these feelings – they may, in some way, be requesting permission to have them – and be comfortable after they have been expressed. Some reassurance may be necessary and valuable, but it should be given carefully, in a nurturing style rather than dictated by an authority figure. Later sessions may explore alternative ways of thinking, feeling or managing the difficulties, and personal abilities. The aim is to encourage parents to hold onto and develop their strengths, although there is a fine line between achieving this aim and encouraging dependency on someone in authority.

I have found that it helps parents who are feeling 'stuck' and depressed to look back with them at what has happened during the past hours, days or weeks. The professional can identify what they have experienced, what has been achieved, as well as what they have achieved personally. For some, it is therapeutic to write feelings down, perhaps to keep a diary, making notes on the child's condition and what was important. Parents usually know their children better than other carers, so what are their observations? What do they feel about them? Consider with them their part in the care, their contributions to the progress, and how strong they have been so far. Reassure them that it is understandable for them to be tired through lack of sleep and worry – anxiety uses up a lot of energy. Suggest that perhaps their bodies are trying to tell them to take some rest and that now might be a good time to do that.

TREATMENT OF DEPRESSION

Riley (1998) summarised treatments for depression into three groups:

- *Drug therapy*, which works on the chemical balance of the brain, includes:
  — tricyclic antidepressants, e.g. amitriptyline, imipramine
  — selective serotonin/noradrenaline reuptake inhibitors, e.g. Prozac
  — monoamine oxidase inhibitors, lithium carbonate (mood stabiliser)
- *Psychological treatments* may be offered alone or in conjunction with drug treatment. They give emotional support while aiming to explore and resolve the cause of the depression and may include:
  — cognitive behavioural therapy
  — psychodynamic psychotherapy/counselling
  — person-centred therapies/counselling.
- *Physical treatments* are rarely used these days except for severely depressed patients. These treatments include:
  — electroconvulsive therapy (ECT) – passing an electric current through the brain to cause a convulsion
  — neurosurgery.

DEPRESSION IN THE SICK CHILD

Children's wards are usually bright and cheerful and every attempt is made to ensure the children are happy, but there may be children resident who are neither happy nor cheerful, and who need to talk about their real feelings and fears. Children often protect their parents from further hurt by concealing certain thoughts and refraining from asking difficult questions.

I have come across older children, who have been ill for a long time or who have had a complicated postoperative recovery, who seem quite unable to move on to a more normal life as they recover physically. Whilst they have been in hospital or sick at home, other people have managed their lives for them – made decisions, waited on them, given them special meals and gifts – and there have been few expectations of them. Making the adjustment, as they get better, to feeling happy and in control of their lives once more, can be extremely difficult. A phase of depression can become a sort of protection, a safety net from the big and frightening world of the fit and active (see Case Study 6.1).

CASE STUDY 6.1 *Refuge in illness*

A teenage girl who was depressed after a prolonged postoperative recovery talked about all the things she wanted to do when she was better, such as going to discos and having a boyfriend, thus giving the impression she did indeed want to get better. She had become dependent on pain-relieving drugs for continuing pain which had no obvious cause. After being treated with antidepressants, she had regular counselling and a spell in hospital for careful withdrawal of the drugs; she was able to be much more positive about herself. She admitted that she had been afraid of being well, of what would be expected of her, so the pain had given her a reason, or excuse, to be ill for longer.

Sometimes a child may need to be allowed to be sad or fed up, at least for a while, and may be helped most by an understanding nurse or helper who listens and agrees that the mood is reasonable in the circumstances. Fears and anxieties might be discussed if a child feels the helper understands, and then appropriate information can be offered to correct any misunderstanding on the part of the child. Continual attempts to cheer up a sick child may, in fact, be counter-productive. As Judd (1989) wrote, referring to a dying child:

An attempt to jolly the child up, to lift him out of his depression, can lead to despair on the part of the child – despair that no one can bear the pain of the loss of the healthy self and the possible loss of life.

One also encounters sick children, particularly if in hospital, who feel bad about being ill. Eiser (1991) suggested that children under 7 years of age tend to believe that illnesses are a punishment for wrongdoing or occur by some magical process.

A child's separation from parents while in hospital can also have an effect on mood which can damage the parent/child relationship. In his now classic film, Robertson (1952) studied a 2-year-old child in hospital. This normal, sociable child was separated from her mother, became gradually withdrawn and then sadly depressed. When the mother returned to visit the child, she was rejected.

As well as the sick child, siblings of sick children have also been known to become depressed. They may believe that they were responsible for the illness of their brother or sister or that they could have prevented it. This type of fantasy, which is common in children in this situation, can lead to depression as the sick child does not get better.

DEPRESSION AMONGST CARERS

Professional carers may also show signs of depression, particularly when they do not seem able to put things right or make them better. Insufficient funding, staff and resources do not help to make the staff feel well supported, especially when managers do not seem to have a real understanding of what is being experienced. Lack of progress or improvement in a patient may lead a doctor or nurse to think they are not doing a good job, and they are rarely praised when they have performed well. Time given to share these thoughts is usually helpful in maintaining morale and confidence.

The families of a child with a serious, life-threatening or chronic illness may have periods of feeling depressed or may need treatment for depression, so health professionals need to be aware of the risks. Other members of the family usually share some of the bad feelings, even if they do not make them known. Health professionals can often empathise with similar feelings and need to have someone of their own to help them reflect on these.

CONCLUSION

Depression remains a complex topic, especially for those working in the field of mental health. It is important for those working with families of sick children to understand the relevance of this subject and to be able to recognise warning signs and offer support and help when needed.

REFERENCES

Beck, A. & Steer, R. (1987) *Beck Depression Inventory Manual*. San Antonio: Harcourt Brace Jovanovitch.

Brown, D. & Pedder, J. (1979) *Introduction to Psychotherapy; an Outline of Psychodynamic Principles and Practice*. London: Tavistock.

Eiser, C. (1991) It's O.K. having asthma ... young children's belief about illness. *Professional Nurse*, **6(6)**, 342–345.

Freud, S. (1917) *Mourning and Melancholia*. London: Pelican Freud Library.

Gibran, K. (1926) *The Prophet*. London: Heinemann.

Jacobs, M. (1986). *The Presenting Past – an Introduction to Practical Psychodynamic Counselling*. London: Harper and Row.

Judd, D. (1989) *Give Sorrow Words – Working with a Dying Child*. London: Free Association Books.

Kübler-Ross, E. (1969) *On Death and Dying*. London: Tavistock/Routledge.

Miller, A. (1987) *The Drama of being a Child*. London: Virago Press.

Noble-Jamieson, G., Cook, P., Parkinson, G. & Barnes, N. (1996) Coping strategies in parents of children receiving liver transplants. *Clinical Child Psychology and Psychiatry*, **1**, 563–573.

Riley, M. (1998) Understanding depression. *Nursing Times*, **94(44)**, 24–27.

Robertson, J. (1952). *A Two Year Old Goes to Hospital* (film). London: Tavistock.

Rycroft, C. (1968) *A Critical Dictionary of Psychoanalysis*. London: Penguin.

Winnicott, D. (1963) *Home is Where We Start From*. London: Pelican.

Loss and separation

INTRODUCTION

Loss and separation are two very important issues for anyone working with sick children. Although the two words are different, they are discussed together in this chapter because in many ways they are similar. It should at least be recognised that there will inevitably be losses associated with separation.

We all experience continual changes in our normal lives, and with these changes come inevitable losses. Some losses are insignificant, while others have deep and lasting effects. Grieving is a natural response to a loss of any kind, and professionals need to understand this and be able to recognise the emotions and feelings that are part of this, rather than be quick to label the parents as 'difficult'. Loss associated with the death of a child is discussed in Chapter 14.

LOSS

The worst fear of parents with a sick child is that of the ultimate loss – the death of the child. For the majority of parents, this represents the loss of their most precious possession, along with the loss of their future hopes and aspirations. The grieving actually begins at the time of the diagnosis; after that, life cannot be the same again, and the hopes for the future change. The child's illness may not be life-threatening, but the parents have become vulnerable and fearful; their stability has been shaken. A natural response to any significant loss is grieving, and this period of mourning a loss has no fixed time limit. It may take parents a surprisingly long time to arrive at an understanding and acceptance of bad news, be it a diagnosis or a poor prognosis, with many and mixed emotions on the way.

Loss of the parent's role as main carer

For the mother and father of a very sick child there may be, even if only temporary, some change in their usual roles. Nurses may need to give the child's feed via a nasogastric tube, and although parents may in time learn to do this themselves, it is not their usual method. Simple everyday activities which they normally perform, such as washing and changing, may be carried out by nurses if the child is in intensive care. It is not surprising that parents say they feel useless and unable to help the child, however much the nurses encourage and help them to do so.

Loss of full responsibility for child

Responsibility for a very sick child has to be shared with professionals when decisions and judgements need to be made in the child's best interest. This highlights the importance of developing an open, honest and trusting relationship at the start, in order to allow parents to feel they are an essential part of the care team, which they should be, and helps to minimise the sense of loss of responsibility.

Decisions should always be taken with the full cooperation and consent of the parents. Health professionals with good counselling skills have a valuable role as a sounding board for parents' thoughts, allowing them time and permission to say what they think and fear, and to confirm their understanding of the situation. It may be helpful for the family to know that critical decisions do not have to be made by them alone; knowing that the medical teams are sharing the responsibility can be a great relief.

Loss of control

Parents may have a sense of loss of control when their child is in hospital; they are to some extent being controlled by the condition of the sick child, and the opinions and advice of the doctors and nurses. They have lost control of events and nothing can be certain. They will be used to having control over normal activities, such as what the child eats and wears, playtimes and bedtimes – much may have changed.

Fear of loss

For some people, feeling out of control brings on unpleasant fears and imaginings and can induce panic. It may revive memories of earlier losses, which can add to the uncertainty, as in Case Study 7.1.

A young baby was admitted to intensive care with bronchiolitis. The baby's mother was very quiet and fidgety; the father felt helpless but was worried about the mother. Watching her sick baby, the mother couldn't help thinking of her first child, who was adopted as part of divorce terms some years ago. That child was taken away from her and she now feared that this one could also be taken away. Compounding her fear of losing her baby was the knowledge that the baby of a close friend had died from the same illness.

Loss of identity

With all the changes which will be going on in their lives and with attention focused on their child, the mother and father may feel they have lost their own identity – they have become 'Matthew's mother' or 'Sasha's father' to the hospital staff. This is particularly true for parents caring for children with chronic and long-term conditions and disabilities, who are kept busy caring for the child and do not continue with their own careers or interests.

When a child is able to go to school or to a centre for special needs, the mothers often have a great need to do something for themselves, almost to prove they can achieve things other than caring for the child. Vicky was one such mother, who was delighted when her child made a good recovery from surgery and was able to return to school. For the last few years, her life had revolved around the child's care and hospital visits and now she felt a strange sense of freedom. She started to study for a degree – something for herself alone. She explained how she would like people to stop her in the street and enquire as to how *she* was, instead of always asking about her child. She wanted to be herself, with her own identity, as well as being her child's mother.

Loss of self-esteem

Children who have a chronic illness and those with physical or mental handicaps may well have precarious self-esteem (Gabell, 1996). They see others who are able to do many things they cannot and often face isolation both practically and as a result of society's attitudes towards them.

During the adolescent years, life is difficult enough for these young people, but having to cope with a chronic condition or disability brings extra problems. Many teenagers will rebel against their condition and refuse to comply with treatment regimes, perhaps secretly destroying medication or eating forbidden foods.

Hair loss from chemotherapy, stomas, amputation, scars and limb abnormalities are but a few examples of changes in body image that may be hard to manage without understanding from adults as well as peers.

Other losses to remember

Any of the losses already discussed can be compounded and complicated by memories and feelings that relate to other events and experiences of loss. These memories may be significant to what is happening now, but just as important are the more common changes that are going on in the family members' lives. These could include illness or death of another family member, loss of employment, moving house, death of a pet, miscarriage, a child changing school or theft; even the car breaking down forces a change in routine activities.

Loss felt by staff

Staff caring for sick children and their families are also affected by losses, which may be frequent and at times overwhelming for those working in intensive care units or with terminally ill children. The effects of constant exposure to such extreme experiences of loss and change are gradually becoming recognised by the nursing profession. Lewis (1998) is convinced that, as individuals and as nurses, it is important to recognise that in any situation our personal feelings will be present:

An ability to cope with loss and change at work is dependent on our individual ability to identify, explore and come to terms with our own feelings so that they may be put aside in order that we can really listen to what others are saying.

SEPARATION

Staff caring for children need to think about the effects that separation has on them and their families. Much importance has been attached to the work in the 1950s and 1960s – in particular that of Robertson (1952) and Bowlby (1969) – concerning the separation anxiety of young children in hospital. Robertson filmed children in hospital and his studies of children before, during and after hospital stays showed that they suffered deep distress at the time and anxiety and insecurity for varying lengths of time after the psychological trauma.

Bowlby (1969) wrote:

...separation in a strange place is known to induce intense distress over a long period, in keeping with Freud's hypothesis that trauma results when the mental apparatus is subjected to excessive quantities of excitation ... it can be demonstrated that the psychological changes that regularly succeed the prolonged distress of separation are none other than: repression, splitting and denial – the defence processes that Freud postulates are the result of trauma.

The strong emotions of love, anxiety, anger and sometimes hatred may all come to be aroused by separation from a single person (Bowlby, 1973):

A period of separation, and also threats of separation and other forms of rejection, are seen as arousing in a child or adult both anxious and angry behaviour. Each is directed towards the attachment figure; anxious attachment is to retain maximum accessibility to the attachment figure; anger is both a reproach at what has happened and a deterrent against it happening again. Thus love, anxiety, anger and sometimes hatred come to be aroused by one and the same person.

Separation from home

A parent who is staying in hospital with a child will be separated from home and the daily routine of managing the family, and perhaps also from work. Resident parents may find it strange to be with that child all day and night, and to be sleeping by the child or in a hospital room. Mothers, in particular, have been heard to say that they miss the housework, and actually find some relaxation from the stress of the ward in washing and ironing the child's clothes; they find relief in doing normal chores. Other parents will miss their work – the company of colleagues, the structure of the day as well as payment.

Separation from partner, family and friends

The parent in hospital can feel quite lonely and isolated from the rest of the family. Separation from the normal support system, be that a partner, a mother or a good friend, is often difficult to bear. However frequently they speak on the telephone, it is not the same. It is often important for parents to have family and friends to visit them, unless the child is very sick in which case it may be too difficult for them.

The siblings may be feeling left out and need to see for themselves what is happening at the hospital. The parent may benefit from time spent with the well child (or children), for reassurance that they are well, and as a reminder of life outside the hospital and the normal routine.

Children in hospital may feel out of contact with their peers, and so might welcome visits from their friends, after school or at weekends. Letters or messages on tape from their class also help the sick child to keep in touch.

Separation from familiar surroundings

A strange environment can be most disturbing for some people and a hospital is full of new and different sights, sounds and smells. Many parents will find the many varied noises of the alarms on monitors and pumps stressful. Fire alarms are tested frequently, but parents and children may need reassurance that they are safe.

Children and adults usually miss their own beds; many units now have bed covers and pillow cases decorated with children's pictures and cartoon characters, which help them to feel at ease. Children in hospital for a long period may be helped by having photographs of their house, family and pets displayed nearby. This will remind them of what they look like and of their continued presence at home.

Robertson and Robertson (1967, 1971) discussed the 'concepts of protest, despair and denial – phases attached to separation from mother when aggravated by strange environment, confinement to cot, multiple caretakers and other stress factors associated with institutional care'. Whenever possible, some time for being held is important for babies, toddlers and older children; this can be done by a nurse or nursery nurse if the parents are not available.

Separation from the child

Even if parents are in hospital with their children, there are times when they may feel separated from them. When a child is unconscious, sedated or on a ventilator, the parents may feel a real loss of contact because they do not get any feedback, such as a smile or physical touch. Every encouragement is offered to enable them to hold a hand, talk to the child, or read a story, whether or not the child can hear them. Parents often talk about 'having their child back again' when they are awake, and about how unbearable it is while they are out of contact.

Another time of separation is when the child is in the operating theatre or other special treatment area. The child is under anaesthesia or sedation and unaware, but the parents are left feeling helpless, knowing that there is nothing they can do for the child during this separation. Parents are usually encouraged to accompany their child to theatre and to stay until the child is anaesthetised, thus avoiding the risk of separating a frightened child from a distressed parent. Many parents stay during resuscitation procedures in accident and emergency departments, but it is important that someone is there to support them and to explain what is happening.

Separation is often thought to be particularly difficult and distressing for mothers. Freud (1930) wrote that the 'communal life of human beings is founded on the compulsion to work and the power of love, ... and [that this] made the woman unwilling to be deprived of the part of herself which had been separated from her – her child'. Fathers may also struggle with strong emotional fears of separation from a sick child. Campbell (1991), writing of his experience as a father of a very sick baby, recalled:

Every day we could see in numbers and coloured lines how her battle for life was being fought. But no matter how ill she was, we found that when we were at her bedside we always felt more reassured than when we were away.

Children visiting an adult in hospital

Whilst we are thinking about children and separation, we should perhaps not forget the needs of children who are separated from a relative or close friend because that person is sick and in hospital. There is a great temptation for well-meaning adults to try to protect a child from hearing bad news, and from seeing unfamiliar or unpleasant sights – in fact, protecting them from reality.

We must consider the child's point of view and the effects on the child. If it is a parent who is in hospital, a mother say, it is likely that the child will be missing her and needing to know where she is, why she is there, who is looking after her and when she is coming home. In this situation, children will also want to know how they can expect to be affected by the parent's absence. If children are not given answers to these questions, they will make up their own. These are unlikely to match the truth of the situation, and will therefore be unhelpful.

If children really do not want to visit, or if it is not advisable, then there are many ways that they can be helped to feel in touch and not left out. Drawing a picture, writing a note, recording a message on tape and choosing flowers are some suggestions. An instant photograph of a parent or sibling in intensive care is often sufficient to allow children to understand why that person cannot be at home, and that he or she is being cared for in a special place where the illness can be treated. Having a photograph to look at when they want, perhaps to take around with them, makes children feel closer and may alleviate their need to see the hospitalised person until there has been some improvement.

CONCLUSION

The effects of separation and loss are sometimes obvious to all, but at other times may not be noticed even by the most experienced of professionals working with families. A loss does not have to mean loss through death; it can mean loss of a role, responsibility, identity, control or self-esteem. There are many everyday losses that are normally important, but which should be acknowledged when a family is struggling with the anxieties of having a sick child. Separation from familiar people, routines, scenery and home and family adds to the sense of chaos and confusion. The world around us is constantly changing, but amidst all this change we are usually able to find some stability and therefore security. However, illness can bring uncertainty and a change of routine and thereby threaten this stability we have constructed around ourselves.

REFERENCES

Bowlby, J. (1969) *Attachment and Loss. Attachment*, vol. 1. London: Hogarth Press.
Bowlby, J. (1973) *Attachment and Loss. Separation, Anxiety and Anger*, vol. 2. London: Hogarth Press.
Campbell, J. (1991) A mystery solved, a life remembered. *The Times*, (London), 4 January 1991.
Freud, S. (1985) *Civilization and its Discontents*, Pelican Freud Library vol. 12. London: Penguin.
Gabell, Y. (1996) Self-esteem and loss. In *Working with Children in Grief and Loss*, ed. Lindsay, B. & Elsegood, J. London: Baillière Tindall.
Lewis, C. (1998) Loss and change on the neonatal intensive care unit. *Paediatric Nursing*, **10(3)**, 21–23.
Robertson, J. (1952) *A Two Year Old Goes to Hospital* (film). London: Tavistock.
Robertson, J. & Robertson, Joyce (1967) *Young Children in Brief Separation* (film). London: Tavistock Child Development Research Unit.
Robertson, J. & Robertson, Joyce (1971) *Young Children in Brief Separation*. NY Times: Quadrangle Books.

FURTHER READING

Bowlby, J. (1964) Attachment. In *Attachment and Loss*, vol. 1: New York: Basic Books.

Bowlby, J. (1980) Loss, sadness and depression. In *Attachment and Loss*, vol. 3. London: Hogarth Press.

Robertson, J. and Robertson, J. (1989) *Separation and the Very Young*. London: Free Association Books.

Using counselling skills to support sick children and their families

INTRODUCTION

The use of the word 'counselling' has extended to include many interpretations which differ from the uses by professional counsellors. These often include issues to do with giving advice and disciplinary procedures. As a trained and practising counsellor, I think of counselling in terms of a therapeutic relationship, where one person helps another. Distinctions must also be made between counselling as a process and the use of counselling skills as part of another professional role, such as nursing, social work or teaching.

Many health professionals are aware of their need to improve these skills, and the availability of short courses continues to increase. Important benefits of learning counselling skills include a heightened self-awareness and feelings of increased confidence to cope with emotions and feelings expressed by others. There are many excellent books on counselling available through bookshops and specialist suppliers, some of which focus on particular fields of work such as bereavement, couples, young people, general practice, crisis and telephone counselling, or victims of trauma and sexual abuse.

This chapter explores some of the issues and benefits of using counselling skills in the context of working with sick children and their families, and the staff caring for them.

WHAT IS MEANT BY COUNSELLING?

The British Association for Counselling (BAC, 1995) uses the following definition in an information sheet:

People become engaged in counselling when a person, occupying regularly or temporarily the role of counsellor, offers or agrees explicitly to offer time, attention and respect to another person or persons temporarily in the role of client.

The task of counselling is to give the client an opportunity to explore, discover and clarify ways of living more resourcefully and towards a greater well-being.

We recognise that two or more counsellors may work together, and that the client may be a single individual or a couple, a family, a group, or a system.

Within the context of working with families, a counsellor may work alone, with a partner or in a team. The client could be a mother or father, a couple, a child or children, a whole family, a group of parents or children, a group of schoolchildren or a staff support group.

Counsellors may work independently or as part of a group of counsellors. They may also be employed by an organisation such as a hospital, health centre, college of health studies or support group. A counsellor might be available by appointment only, or might be an active member of a multidisciplinary team. It is often easier to talk to counsellors if they are provided as part of the care team. Psychological support is recognised to be sufficiently important when someone is employed for that purpose. Parents have reported that it was helpful to know that other parents also needed support and that they were not the only ones to feel they needed help to cope with their situation.

AIMS OF COUNSELLING

The main aim must surely be to help, and in the context of sick children and their families, one needs to ask:

- *What might help?* Regular opportunities to talk about problems and how they are managing them and what they are thinking and feeling. Knowing that there is someone they can contact who is available to listen to them, who will understand, especially when the sick child's condition changes or the family has added problems.
- *Who might help?* Possibly someone in the health care team, social services, or a counsellor.
- *How might the client be helped?* By being offered time and attention to enable them to explore their feelings and fears. A counselling role can be very supportive alongside the medical and nursing care of the child.

Counselling is essentially a helping and supporting relationship where one person is there to help another. It is more than a friendship or befriending and no advice or practical help is offered.

The counsellor aims to enable clients to explore problems by acknowledging the realities of the situation – what they really mean, from their point of view, including the real difficulties, anxieties and feelings, both good and bad. By good listening and reflecting, the counsellor may help clients to find alternative ways of thinking and feeling.

The supportive element in counselling is vital to initial 'survival' and subsequent personal growth of the person being helped. The counsellor has a holding and nurturing role that aims to reinforce that person's ways of coping, perhaps building on past experience. There is also a need to monitor the levels of reality, balancing what is or is not achievable and perhaps helping the person to come to terms with the truth of a situation. This is sometimes essential for parents of a child who is critically or chronically sick.

THE COUNSELLING PROCESS OR USING COUNSELLING SKILLS?

A distinction must be drawn between:

- professional counselling and the counselling process
- counselling skills and their use within many other roles and professions.

People who practise as counsellors should have completed a reputable course of training that includes theory and practice, with experience of being counselled and counselling with supervision. There are many methods, models and styles but they all share similar aims of helping clients to help themselves.

Counsellors offer regular sessions, usually weekly for an hour. This may continue for any length of time, from a few sessions to several years of therapy. Counselling concentrates on the person with the problems, rather than on the actual problems. During this time clients work through their difficulties, explore their feelings and thoughts and hopefully achieve a more fulfilling life, with a better understanding of themselves and the world around them. This process of change, with the methods and techniques used by the counsellor, is often referred to as *the counselling process*.

Tschudin (1995) described this process of helping and caring effectively as a flow, or movement forwards, from problem to goal, from dissatisfaction to satisfaction, from being stuck to resourcefulness. Tschudin identified four stages:

1. To define the starting point and clarify the problem
2. To gain some insight into why there is a problem
3. To discover a goal to aim for
4. To explore the ways and means of getting there.

Nelson-Jones (1993) introduced a five-stage lifeskills helping model – DASIE – as follows:

D   – develop the relationship, identify and clarify problems
A   – assess problem(s) and redefine in skills terms
S   – state working goals and plan interventions
I   – intervene to develop self-helping skills
E   – end and consolidate self-helping skills.

Counselling skills are those used by counsellors, but they are also used by many others in their work with people. The difference is that people who are temporarily in the role of client may not be seeking counselling as such, but are helped considerably by these skills. Awareness and practised use of these skills can be of great assistance to health professionals who need to be able to deal with difficult situations involving patients, families and themselves. Training in counselling skills is not, on its own, sufficient for users to consider themselves as qualified counsellors (BAC, 1989). However, nurses who have undertaken counselling skills courses usually find that their coping methods and self-confidence are boosted.

ESSENTIAL PERSONAL QUALITIES OF A COUNSELLOR

The only tools of this trade are those you keep with you at all times – you as a person and your skills and experiences. It is therefore very important that helpers are aware of their own personalities and characteristics. It is important, too, for clients to be able to decide for themselves whether or not a counsellor is suitable for them.

It might be useful to think of someone known to you, who is good to talk to, and to ask yourself why you find it easy to talk to that person. Make a list of the good qualities and then think of someone you could not talk to and list the reasons why. After asking many people to do this myself, I obtained a variety of positive and negative qualities, and these are listed in Box 8.1. I am sure there are many more words and phrases that could be added to this box, but those listed do show some of the feelings as to what is important in a person who is offering help. Carl Rogers (1961) noted, from studies of helping relationships, 'that

---

Box 8.1   Positive and negative human qualities as identified by a number of responders

Positive qualities

- Helpful
- Able to reduce stress
- Sense of humour
- Knows limitations
- Able to act as a go-between
- Rewarding
- Provider
- Self-aware
- Smiling face
- Caring
- Good telephone communication
- Not easily shocked
- Perceptive
- Well balanced
- Relieve anxiety
- Accepting
- Sincere

- Understanding
- Good listener
- Able to break down barriers
- Confidential
- Trust
- Confident in own ability
- Non-judgemental
- Gentle
- Non-threatening
- Softly spoken
- Stable personality
- Interpreter of body language
- Impartial
- Gives time
- Reliable
- Open

- Interested
- Honest
- Supportive
- Strong
- Warm
- Empathy
- Patient
- Approachable
- Calm
- Good memory
- Mature
- Not involved
- Relaxed
- Good role model
- Genuine
- Consistent

Negative qualities

- Impatient
- Easily distracted
- Gossips
- A 'know it all'
- Stares into eyes
- Gives advice
- Poor positioning of seats
- Too intense
- Uncaring
- Inappropriate reflection
- Extreme dress or appearance
- No smiles
- Changes mind

- Fidgets
- Interrupts
- Too forceful
- Forgetful
- Judgmental
- Finishes sentences for speaker
- Pressure of time
- 'Nosey'
- Lack of privacy
- Controlling
- Loud voice, noisy
- Writes notes
- Insincere

- Bad habits (e.g. picks nose, sniffs)
- Intrusions (including noises, smells)
- Says 'I know how you feel'
- No eye contact
- Talks too much
- Not interested
- Talks about self
- Too much sympathy
- Negative body language
- Too directive
- Monotonous voice
- Unreliable

---

it is the attitudes and feelings of the therapist, rather than his theoretical orientation, which is important. His procedures and techniques are less important than his attitudes'.

Concerning the nurse in the role of helper, Scholes (1996) made some useful research observations:

The notion of the nurse's presence having a therapeutic or anti-therapeutic effect has been recorded by Ersser (1991) and has been explored as a concept of intimacy or closeness by Savage (1995). They found that the presence of the nurse and how she presented to the patient was as important as the task she was performing.

Other factors that may be important for the client when considering seeing a counsellor are listed in Box 8.2.

Box 8.2   Factors to consider in a counsellor

Positive qualities
- Age
- Sexual orientation
- Colour
- Language spoken
- Convenience of meetings
- Social status – married, single, divorced, widowed, parent,
- Type of counselling available
- Location of the sessions

- Gender
- Race
- Lifestyle
- Religious beliefs
- Cost

Counsellors should also think about personal issues that may determine whether they would be suitable for a particular client. Following a recent death in the family, a counsellor might decide that it would be unwise to offer bereavement counselling to someone else, at least for a while.

Counsellors must be open and accepting to what clients bring to a session, and so should be aware of their own raw feelings and emotions as well as their personal values, morals and prejudices.

THE IMPORTANCE OF SELF-AWARENESS AND PERSONAL SURVIVAL

It cannot be emphasised strongly enough that counselling can be emotionally draining for the therapist. It is a privileged and humbling role to be entrusted with a great deal of very personal and private information. Sometimes counsellors may feel vulnerable when issues are raised which 'touch a raw nerve' for them. It is therefore with good understanding of the subject that I choose to consider personal survival and self-awareness together. Counsellors must aim to survive, despite what might be thrown at them. It is vital to this survival that they know themselves well enough to understand what makes them vulnerable, that they know their strengths and weaknesses, and that they have discovered what helps them to cope and how they can relax and 'switch off' from their work. All of this is equally important for anyone working in the caring professions.

Those who work with families often become very involved with them, especially with children. It is sometimes hard for nurses caring for a sick child to be able to erect boundaries between their work and their time off. Strong bonds may grow, particularly if a nurse is a child's special nurse. The child may be dependent on the nurse for good care and perhaps fun and affection while in hospital, but at the same time the child could be fulfilling the nurse's need to be wanted and to be reassured that he is, indeed, a good nurse.

It is not difficult to understand how a nurse might want to continue pleasing a family and might be reluctant, almost to the point of possessiveness, to allow others to take over this role. So the less experienced nurse may start to come in to visit the child on days off, or perhaps take a parent to the shops or out for tea. This is done with the best of intentions, out of a genuine wish to help, and with kindness. But what does this do to the relationship between the nurse and the family? It changes it from a professional and therapeutic one to a friendship, and these are very different. The boundaries have been moved, which can lead to insecurity on both sides.

The issue of boundaries is therefore an important one for the helper's personal survival, and it is quite likely that someone else will observe the warning signs and encourage the helper to be aware of and talk about what is happening. I agree with Stewart (1979), who wrote:

Over-involvement is painful and calls for a radical reappraisal of our attitudes, emotions and responses to other people. If we have an understanding mentor who is skilled in counselling, then we can turn over-involvement into a positive learning experience.

This emphasises the valuable support of good supervision.

Case Study 8.1 describes a young nurse who was not aware of how deeply involved, emotionally, she had become with her patient, and who felt at risk of not surviving the situation. Jacobs (1986) emphasised that

...it is through becoming aware of their own needs that, paradoxically, people are able to care better for others; treating them not as persons on whom their own needs are projected, but as people in their own right.

Brown and Pedder (1979) also stated that: 'Coming to terms with oneself and learning through experience are part of the psychotherapeutic process for therapists as well as for patients'.

Rogers (1961) wrote much about the importance of being honest with yourself, of knowing yourself and trusting your own intuition as your most reliable guide. It is only when people can be accepting of themselves that they can begin to accept others whom they seek to help. We need to know our own morals, prejudices and values, but also to remember that they are ours and not expect them to be the same for everyone.

CASE STUDY 8.1   *Blurring of the work/home boundary*

Alison was a young nurse who really loved working with children. She became very attached to a little girl who had been on the ward for several weeks, and knew her family. The grandmother had given her a photograph of the child because she knew she was fond of her.

Alison was very distressed at seeing the child in intensive care following major surgery. She admitted that she had not been able to sleep the night before the operation, as she was so anxious. The girl's photograph was by her bed at home and she could not get her out of her mind. Alison commented that the other nurses seemed to be coping much better with the situation than she was.

We talked about the boundaries between time at work and time away from the hospital. She was able to realise that work had invaded her private space; the child belonged to her work time but the photograph had brought her right home to her own bedside. We discussed the issues around where her responsibilities for this child really ended. She agreed that this child was not hers; she was only involved with her in a professional role. How she performed that role was clearly important for her and for the child and her family.

Tschudin (1995) stressed the vital importance of genuineness: 'Only when you are not trying to be "somebody" but are simply yourself can you be trustworthy, dependable and consistent, and only then will you be seen as such by the client'. Parents of sick children need honesty, not only in the information given to them but also in the personalities of those who give it and who try to help them.

COUNSELLING SKILLS

These are the skills used in formal counselling, but they are also used by others who help people to manage their problems. They 'enhance the performance of a functional role, as line manager, nurse, tutor, social worker, personnel officer, voluntary worker and the recipient will in turn, perceive them in that role' (BAC, 1989). Counselling is about building a therapeutic relationship between two people, so it is not surprising that most of the skills are concerned with *listening* and *responding* (see Box 8.3).

Box 8.3   Counselling skills – listening and responding

- Giving attention
- Paraphrasing
- Reflecting feelings
- Communicating understanding
- Clarifying
- Summarising
- Empowering
- Focusing
- Evaluating
- Exploring
- Allowing
- Goal setting

Listening

It is often surprising to discover just how difficult it can be to listen effectively. The short exercise below can be tried with a friend or colleague and may help to highlight some of the difficulties.

Exercise

In pairs, one partner talks to the other for 3 minutes about a chosen topic. The listener must not interrupt, but must try to remember what has been said.

After the set time, the listener repeats back to the speaker what was said. The speaker then becomes the listener for 3 minutes while the partner remembers and repeats what was said.

This exercise may appear easy, but there is much to learn from it. Here are a few thoughts:

As a speaker

- How did it feel to have someone sitting with you, just listening to what you said?
- It may have felt uncomfortable, especially as it was an exercise, so how important was the attitude of the listener?
- Did you think about the listener and want to make what you said interesting or easy to remember?
- Were you able to talk about personal matters?
- Did you have difficulty speaking for the set time, even though it was only 3 minutes? Could you tolerate pauses or did you feel you must continue talking?

As a listener

- Could you resist the urge to join in the conversation, or were you able to just listen?
- How easy was it to remember what was said?
- Did you tolerate any pauses or silences, or did you feel you had to fill the gaps because it was uncomfortable?
- Were you able to pick up feelings behind what was being said?
- Did you notice the speaker's body language? How did it fit with what was being said?
- Was anything said which aroused feelings in you?

The following quote is from someone who writes with the experience of listening to people who need to talk, as well as having had her own need to talk during difficult periods in her life (Spufford, 1989):

People who seek one out in trouble are most helped by attentive silence, into which they can speak, assured of compassion. Any personal reflection of one's own is almost always destructive or disruptive.

Spufford expresses very simply, but accurately, the value of listening in a helping relationship. This must be reassuring for the inexperienced helper who may feel inadequately prepared to help someone in trouble.

Many writers have described the essential elements in a good counselling relationship as genuineness, warmth and empathy. Without these, people would not feel able to speak about their problems, so they must be present before the listening can begin.

Training courses in counselling should include some experience of being counselled, as well as counselling others, with good supervision. This helps the counsellor to understand a little of what it is like to talk to someone who is willing to listen, which is important in building empathy in a therapeutic relationship. Nurses and other professionals may be keen to join in, rather than keeping quiet and listening. In their work, they give advice and 'make better' and it is not always a natural reaction to be non-directive and to be guided by the person they are trying to help.

Responding

After the active listening, responding may involve some, if not most, of the skills listed in Box 8.3. The listener's response is the opportunity to summarise what has been heard and to reflect the feelings behind what was said. The listener should always be tentative, as they could have picked up the wrong message, and this is a chance to clarify the facts. Appropriate responses might give permission to express strong feelings, to allow someone to feel the way they do and to explore difficult issues. The listener may be able to focus on particular thoughts or problems and set some realistic goals.

Many people willing to help may find that they do not know what to say; they have listened to what someone has told them but are afraid of giving the wrong reply. Situations like this often arise, and in this case, it is perhaps best simply to listen for the feelings behind what is being said and to acknowledge them. This makes an immediate link with the person and demonstrates an understanding of their situation.

The same difficulties may arise when someone does not speak, as, for example, in the case of a mother who has been up all night with her sick child and who is sitting silently by the bed, yawning and staring out of the window. It is often helpful to interrupt the silence, just to be friendly, to start a conversation before giving information about the child or to give encouragement to the mother to talk about how she feels. It may, for example, help to sit beside her and to say something like: 'I hear you had a rough time last night, you must be so tired now.'

Interpreting non-verbal clues

Watching the body language of someone who is speaking may add considerably to the overall interpretation of what is being said. The listener might be able to pick out certain actions that could be significant. Clues may also be gleaned from observing people's general appearance, how they hold themselves or sit and move about, the tone and strength of their voice, and their facial expression and eye movements (see Case Studies 8.2 and 8.3).

CASE STUDY 8.2   Non-verbal clues in an adult

The grandmother of a sick child was very tearful and wanted some time to talk about her anxious feelings. She was holding a tissue that had become quite wet from drying her tears and as she spoke, she teased the tissue into little pieces. The pieces were rolled between her thumb and fingers and as tiny strands broke away, they fell to the floor. The distraught lady did not seem to be aware of what she was doing as she told her story. When she stood up to go, she looked down and said: 'Oh what a mess!' I felt it appropriate to comment that perhaps that was how life seemed to her at present – a mess, her normal life had been torn to shreds around her.

CASE STUDY 8.3   Non-verbal expression in a child

Mandy did not want to be at the hospital. Her aunt had insisted that she come with her to see her brother who was seriously injured after being knocked over by a car. Their parents were already at his bedside.

Mandy sat outside the ward, in the corner of a waiting room, alone. She had pulled the cuffs of her jumper right down over her hands and the neck up over her nose, and had her chin on her chest. She gave the impression of trying to be invisible and would not look up when anyone spoke to her.

It was quite obvious that Mandy did not want to talk; she did not want to be there. This girl had witnessed the accident and was probably feeling guilty that she may have caused it because of the argument she had had with her brother immediately before he started to cross the road. It seemed important to help her acknowledge this and to try to imagine how she was feeling; otherwise she would become more isolated and frightened.

I sat down near her and introduced myself as someone who talked with children, and said that I would like to help her. She sat motionless, still looking at the floor, until I said: 'This must be terrible for you, too terrible to talk about.' Then she nodded her head slowly, without looking up. I went on to say that I guessed she was feeling that she might have caused the accident, and that no matter who told her that it was not her fault, she would not believe them. Mandy nodded again with long slow nods. I explained what the doctors had told her parents about her brother's condition, because she was important enough to know too. I said that she did not have to go in to see him if she did not want to, but that we would help her if she would like to.

Mandy did not speak during my time alone with her, but the nodding and shaking of her head became very expressive. I felt that I had been able to break through her isolation by helping her to feel we were trying to understand her awful situation. A short while later, her grandfather asked her to hold his hand as he was rather afraid and would like her to go in with him. She went to see her brother and his nurse welcomed her warmly.

STYLES OF COUNSELLING

There are many schools of training and thought in the field of counselling and psychotherapy; in the context of supporting families of sick children, it is fair to suggest that most approaches are suitable. If we think of counselling in this context as being mainly supportive in aim, it is helpful to consider Winnicott's (1986) thoughts about 'holding'. He uses the word 'holding' to mean a practical application of care-cure rather than remedy-cure:

What we have done is to facilitate growth, not to apply a remedy. We cannot cure a mother of her anxieties about her sick child, but counselling may help her to find her own personal solution or way of managing emotional difficulties, communication problems and interpersonal relationships.

So much of support is about helping to hold a distressed person, both physically and emotionally. The old saying, 'a trouble shared is a trouble halved' highlights that the burden of problems can be lightened by talking about them, by someone else helping to hold them.

Let us explore Winnicott's thoughts on 'holding' a little more. He refers frequently to the 'nursing triad' in relation to a new mother's need to be held emotionally while she holds the baby (Winnicott, 1958). He recognised the mother's need to be believed in, as a 'good enough mother'. After many years in the nursing profession, I know that nurses need holding too, while they hold the patient. They also need reassurance and encouragement to believe in themselves as a 'good enough' nurse.

Winnicott talks about this mother–baby relationship a great deal in his writings – 'acts of human reliability make communication long before speech means anything' – and considers that our belief and subsequent trust in people will develop if we are started off well by 'good enough' parenting. For the parents of sick children, there is enormous dependence on the reliability of the caring team, just as children depend on their parents. Winnicott recognised this responsibility when, as a paediatrician, he wrote: 'One cannot help becoming a parent figure when one is doing anything professionally reliable'.

So which style of counselling is favoured for working with sick children and families? There is no simple answer to this question, as much depends on the experience of the helper and the individual circumstances of the person being helped. Living and working with sick children can be very stressful and exhausting, so worries about conforming to specific counselling methods and models should not be added to the existing pressures. Good active listening with appropriate responses remain the fundamental elements in helping children and their families.

Professionals usually have many facets to their working role and may meet a family in different places – hospital, school, home, clinic, even in a corridor or car park. Responding to the needs of the person in front of you is what is important and this should not be forgotten. In this way, counsellors probably use many methods and models, adapting them according to the needs of the situation. A few of them are described below. A background knowledge of some counselling theory provides a valuable base on which to build experience.

Person-centred counselling

Carl Rogers, an American psychologist, used the term 'counselling' instead of psychotherapy. His book *Client Centred Therapy* was published in 1951 and, as Thorne (1984) noted, it was with this publication 'that he became a major force in the world of psychotherapy, and established his position as a practitioner, theorist and researcher who warranted respect'.

In another of his books, Rogers (1961) described in detail his experiences and feelings about helping others. He believed that everyone, even the most distressed and disturbed, had within themselves the ability to help themselves to grow and develop in a positive direction. This belief is worth remembering, as it can give support and hope to those working with desperately distressed parents of sick children. Rather than treating or trying to cure a person, Rogers (1961) realised that 'change appears to come about through experience in a relationship'. This 'relationship' was the key to success and he emphasised the importance of the following core elements:

- *Being genuine* – in the relationship and with yourself. 'It is only by providing the genuine reality which is in me, that the other person can successfully seek for the reality in him. It seems extremely important to be real' (Rogers, 1961). Genuineness is related to honesty, both of which are vital in building trust. A trusting relationship is important in any situation where one person tries to help another.
- *Acceptance* – Rogers (1961) described acceptance of a client as having 'a warm regard for him as a person of unconditional self worth – of value no matter what his condition, his behaviour, or his feelings'. Acceptance also involves trying to understand the person, and making a safe relationship in which that person has the freedom to explore feelings, free from threatening judgements.
- *Empathy* – Rogers extends his acceptance of a person to include 'a deep empathic understanding which enables me to see his private world through his eyes'. He sees himself as a companion to his client, as he feels free to search for himself. Therapists must be secure in their own identity and understand their own feelings before they can take the risk of being overwhelmed by the client's troubled world.

Person-centred counselling is a gentle, non-threatening and non-directive way of helping, which makes it a good approach for families with a sick child. Rogers (1961) maintained that the outcome of this helping relationship was for clients to be able to find within themselves the tendency 'upon which all psychotherapy depends – the urge to expand, extend, become autonomous, develop, mature, express and activate all the capacities of the self'. In the context of sick children, person-centred counselling helps individuals who are struggling to survive the anxiety, fear and stresses of having a sick child to find the strength and the means to manage within themselves. Having a companion on this journey is extremely supportive.

Pschodynamic counselling

A more dynamic method is sometimes needed, especially if the client is hoping to make major changes in the way of thinking, or if the psychological history has been complex. Our past experiences play a large part in our present behaviour. As Brown and

Pedder (1979) wrote: 'The present can only be understood in terms of the past. The past is ever present.'

Psychodynamic counsellors adopt 'a quiet reflective style, intervening when the client is ready to make use of a particular interpretation' (Brown and Pedder, 1979). This is particularly significant when working with the parents of sick children, as they are often too distressed to be able to respond to interpretations and interventions. The relationship between client and therapist is significant; the counsellor works to interpret the transference (the way the client sees the therapist) and the counter-transference (the feelings the client arouses in the therapist).

The 'triangle of insight' is a term used by psychotherapists and counsellors who work psychodynamically. The three points of the triangle are:

- past relationships, feelings and events
- present relationships, feelings and events in the everyday life of the client
- the relationship between the therapist and the client, including the reactions and feelings that arise within it.

Most people who work to help others do not have a lengthy training in psychotherapy, but I mention those three points here to emphasise their importance and their relevance to a helping relationship.

Many parents with a sick child will have had difficult periods in their previous life history, which may add to their present vulnerability. These could include, among many others, problems with relationships, traumatic events, bad memories and unresolved grief.

Short-term counselling

Individuals who seek help do not always have sufficient time, money or available counsellors to enter a long period of counselling, but there are alternatives. Many GP surgeries now offer counselling sessions for their patients, either by employing counsellors in the practice or by referring patients to a counsellor. Patients are usually offered an initial four or six sessions. In some areas, there are also 'drop-in' centres where people can see a counsellor once or for a few sessions.

This type of help requires the counsellor to work within a time frame and to focus on particular issues, possibly negotiating with the client to work only with what can be managed. A few questions may help, such as:

- Why have you come?
- Why now?
- What are the problems?
- How did they start?
- What are your expectations?

Counsellors working in hospitals are often asked to undertake this type of counselling: they may only see a client for one or several sessions, which may last for a few minutes or for an hour or more. If further sessions are needed, they can be arranged as appropriate.

Preparing for an event

Case Study 8.4 illustrates how a short counselling session can help to prepare parents of a sick child for a difficult event or experience, in this case the terrible reality of the forthcoming death of their child. Active planning is a necessary part of how we will cope with unfamiliar situations and counselling will certainly help to explore fears and expectations. It is important in many, if not most, fields of work with sick children and families – sometimes preparing the child separately or preparing the parents to help the child.

CASE STUDY 8.4   Short-term counselling in hospital – preparing for a death

A young couple asked to see me as there were a few problems they wanted to discuss. Their only child suffered from a degenerative condition for which there was no cure. He was obviously deteriorating quite quickly and they were realising that he could die sooner than they had thought. This was frightening for them, but they were determined to care for him at home, giving him all the love they could while he was with them. A paediatric community nurse made regular visits and was available whenever they needed help, and the parents felt well supported by an excellent nurse.

The difficulty for the parents arose in actually thinking about the moment of his death. They felt desperately guilty – because his condition was genetically determined, but also for thinking about his death while he was still alive. They were finding it hard to accept the nurse's suggestion of a nasogastric tube for feeding him, even though he was not able to swallow properly anymore, as they regarded that as failing their son.

We talked about the tube feeding, and how it would remove the risk of choking. They would learn how to pass the tube and care for it, and give him his milk from a syringe instead of a bottle. Although this was not the way they had been used to feeding him, they would be making him comfortable by satisfying his hunger more successfully than persisting with a teat which he could not suck. This chat helped them to realise that while their need was to feed him as normal by bottle, his need was to have his hunger satisfied, and that it did not matter to him how this was done.

> Being unable to feed was another stage closer to death, and this was the parents' greatest dread. We talked about this for some time; they were very realistic, yet seeking permission to let him go when the time came. They were able to say what they would find most difficult and we 'rehearsed' what might happen. They agreed to stay calm, that there was no need to panic and call the emergency services; instead they could cuddle him and quietly call the GP and nurse.
>
> This couple found great relief in facing what was inevitable but still unthinkable. In relative safety and privacy, we spent just over an hour breaking down their fears and defences, strengthening their own ways of coping and their devotion to the child and to each other.
>
> In a strange way, I felt proud of them when they told me, a few weeks later, that the child had died peacefully in their arms, and that they had been pleased to have given him a dignified death at home with them as they wished.

Our self-conceptions help us to stabilise our anticipation of events. If we think we are good at a task, then we will expect to do it well, and if we are familiar with a route, we are unlikely to get lost. Hence, previous knowledge of a situation we face can be reassuring, if our earlier experience was positive. However, it is also true that a previous negative experience can cause anxiety when faced with the situation once more.

The psychologist Kelly (1991) described human future orientation in his theory of personal constructs: 'a person's processes are psychologically channelled by the ways in which he anticipates events'. This theory is based 'on the premise that the essential characteristic of people is that they construct models in order to anticipate events' (Cunningham and Davis, 1985). If there is no model, then we make one up in order to make sense of events and possible alternatives. If the model we create is incorrect, our expectations will not be fulfilled, which leads to anger at the model going wrong or at our inability to cope without one. The conflicts and confusion that arise need to be explored to see where the model does not fit with what is actually happening.

Personal construct theory maintains that there are alternative ways of looking at any event (Stewart, 1997), but does not pay much attention to feelings, which are necessary considerations when working with families of sick children. It is therefore not very useful as a means of helping them, but highlights the importance of preparing for events in order to cope.

How we think ahead and imagine or visualise the features of a future event plays a significant role in how we cope with the situation when it arises. This 'preplanning' may restrict the individual somewhat, a kind of 'tunnel vision', and time may be needed to undo the preconditioning and allow a more realistic understanding. The threat of the whole truth may force people into an unconscious narrowing of their perceptions, so that they concentrate only on selected areas, whereas a much broader perspective would enable them to take in more information and give them more options upon which to act.

One mother said that the very phrase 'intensive care' conjured up a frightening picture – 'a chamber of horrors' was how she imagined it. After her child's stay in the unit she spoke of the wonderful air of hope, joy and love which she had felt in there.

It does, therefore, seem right that, whenever possible, time should be spent with parents before they are in the intensive care unit with their child, or indeed prior to any new experience or event. They need to be given the facts about their child's condition and why they need particular treatment – what will happen, what they will see and what they can do for their child – before their imaginations construct inaccurate pictures. Unhurried attention for them at this stage also gives an opportunity to express fears and preconceived ideas (see Case Study 8.5).

CASE STUDY 8.5 Preconceptions can be damaging

The mother of a very sick child could barely speak, but was able to say how she had focused on her child's ashen skin colour. All she could think of was 'the colour' and, given time, she told me how the awful memory came to her of seeing her mother turn that same colour after her death only 3 months previously. She was extremely worried that her child was going to die, because the colour was such a powerful reminder.

Professionals should always be sensitive to a child's need for honest information; they need correct building blocks to construct their images of what is going to happen; otherwise they will build their own, based on fantasy rather than on the truth, which may be highly damaging.

Confrontation may be used to draw attention deliberately to issues being avoided, and will, hopefully, encourage honesty in expressing thoughts and feelings. An example of this is when a parent is refusing to consider the possibility that her child might die. This is understandable; she does not want to hear it, even less to have to believe it. The doctors may arrange a meeting with the parents for the purpose of addressing the issue, as discussion about future treatment could not progress until they acknowledged this fact.

Gestalt therapy

Some methods used in gestalt therapy (Page, 1984; Stewart, 1997) may be helpful in situations such as that described above, but gestalt therapy training is lengthy (see Case Study 8.6). Gestalt therapists work in the present, with what is in front of them, believing that 'a person lives in the present and can only experience, respond, feel and think in the here and now: change only occurs in the present' (Page, 1984). The mother in Case Study 8.6 was able to act out in the present what she was experiencing at that moment and this proved to be very helpful.

CASE STUDY 8.6 *The gestalt approach*

A mother found that she could not talk to the doctors on the ward and would rush outside when they came in, because she did not want them to give her bad news. We sat down and talked about what she meant by 'bad news'. Eventually she was able to act out a conversation with the doctor by playing his role, in which he would tell her the worst things she could hear. This turned out to be incredibly important as she had been under a complete misunderstanding about her child's condition. We were able to dispel her worst fears and after that she was encouraged to speak with the doctors herself. As her self-confidence grew, she became much more interested in the care of her child and of herself and her appearance.

Sometimes, when I have sensed strong anger in someone, for example, I have used the 'empty chair' technique to enable them to let the feelings out. The client imagines that the person with whom they are angry is sitting in the empty chair in front of them and says what they want to say to them, as did the mother in Case Study 8.6. The client can change chairs in order to give a reply. Hitting a pillow may also be helpful in releasing pent-up anger. Gestalt therapy works on unresolved feelings or unfinished business, and so encourages the letting go of feelings, aiming for a 'whole' or 'complete' person.

Crisis counselling

A crisis for one person may not be a crisis for another; a great deal will depend on the temperament of an individual, previous ability to cope, the reality and risk of the situation, the available resources and support, and other personal factors. The term crisis is usually used to represent a temporary period when someone is unable to 'cope' with a threatening situation. According to Kfir (1989), in a crisis 'information is lacking, support is insufficient, alternatives are hidden'. Kfir's approach to crisis intervention is to address these factors by obtaining and giving information, offering support and providing alternatives.

This may sound simple enough; a person in crisis needs everything simplified to help make life manageable. What is needed most is emotional rescue and first aid help – immediately. This offers a lifeline to hold on to, to prevent drowning in the sea of confusion and panic. A crisis is a new but unexpected experience for which we are unprepared and therefore we do not know how to deal with our reactions. A crisis is not a disaster; it forces us to develop new responses and ways of coping, so the aim must be not only to survive a crisis, but also to grow and develop from the experience.

Wright (1986) divided crises into two types:

- coincidental – sudden illness, accident, redundancy, loss of income, loss of status, loss of security, divorce/separation
- developmental – birth, puberty/adolescence, courtship, marriage, pregnancy, menopause, death.

Sudden death fits both categories.

There are many possible crises for families of sick children and it is understandable that professionals may feel paralysed by an overwhelming situation. Being with a distressed person and trying to be a good listener are helpful; the situation is likely to be more bearable if the person is not alone, but that may not be enough. The person in crisis may be 'disabled' and may need a helper to intervene. The enormity of the crisis may be too much to think about, especially in the early stages, so giving the person the most important piece of information or dealing with an immediate problem and contacting someone who can give support may provide the necessary lifetime. Giving the person just one small task that she can manage will help her to maintain some confidence in her ability to survive.

Post-trauma counselling

In the context of this book, it is not appropriate to discuss counselling offered to victims, survivors and helpers after major disasters, but on a small scale, a traumatic event with a sick child could be considered a major disaster for that family. Parents may be able to stay relatively calm after being given bad news or find the energy to stay awake all night while their child needs emergency surgery, but they may need some help to work through some of the feelings afterwards. Parents who have been through an anxious period with a child in the intensive care unit often find it helpful to talk about their experiences when the child is able to go to a ward. It is as if it is not safe to let go of the feelings until the child is better (see Case Study 8.7).

CASE STUDY 8.7   Post-trauma counselling

A mother asked a ward nurse if her 13-year-old son could have counselling as he was having nightmares and flashbacks following his accident a week ago. Craig was knocked off his bicycle while he was delivering newspapers, and had sustained a minor head injury and fractured leg.

He told me the story of his accident in his own words, starting with delivering the papers and ending with his memories of being in hospital. I then asked him about the flashbacks and nightmares and they always took him to the same place in the story – when he was lying on the road. We talked about what it was like – what he saw, felt, did and thought. That was his worst moment of the trauma as he had been extremely afraid that no one would come and save him. We moved on to what happened next – who came, what did they look like, what did they do and what did they say?

Craig remembered that a 'nice lady' bent down to talk to him; she was smiling and had a gentle voice. A car driver stopped and called an ambulance on his mobile phone and put his jacket over him. He remembered hearing the ambulance siren and I asked him how that made him feel. He smiled and said he knew then he would be alright. The ambulance men told him jokes on the way to hospital.

We returned to discuss the flashbacks and made a plan: whenever he remembered the horror of lying in the road and feeling afraid, he was to think about the nice lady with the smiling face, then the man with the mobile phone, and then how it felt to hear the ambulance coming. All those kind people did come to save him. He had learned a way of helping himself to move on from bad to good memories. A few days later, his mother reported that he was sleeping better and not getting the flashbacks.

SUPERVISION AND SUPPORT

Counselling supervision/consultative support refers to a formal arrangement which enables counsellors to discuss their counselling regularly with one or more people who have an understanding of counselling and counselling supervision/consultative support (BAC, 1996). The British Association for Counselling recommends that all counsellors should have regular supervision.

Clinical supervision is available for many health professionals, including nurses, social workers and psychologists. It offers similar support, both in their clinical work and in reflecting on their use of counselling skills.

REFERRING ON TO OTHER AGENCIES

Helpers must realise when a person needs specialised help beyond what they are able to offer. In other words, know when you are out of your depth, because if you are floundering, so will the person you are trying to help.

There are many organisations offering specific help, such as for couples, bereavement, homosexuals and lesbians, drugs and alcohol abuse. The client may need medical help such as medication for insomnia or depression, or may need to consult a psychiatrist or psychologist. Some families have long-term problems coping with an illness, bereavement or trauma. Departments such as Child and Family Consultation Clinics offer help to parents and children, as either individual or family therapy. Special clinics are available for children who have witnessed violence or other traumatic events.

CONCLUSION

At the end of this chapter, I would like to return to where we began, and remember that counselling and using counselling skills are about helping. There are many models and ways of working and even more books and articles from which to learn the theory on which to base your practice.

Tschudin (1995) provided guidelines for helping in the form of 'four questions'. They make an excellent model that keeps the focus on the client, and can be used either for a brief session or for long-term therapy. They can be a useful framework and offer a summary for working with families of sick children:

1. *What is happening?* What is going on here? What is the person saying or not saying? What is going on between us (client and helper)? What am I hearing? What am I not hearing?
2. *What is the meaning of it?* What significance does the problem have in the client's life? What memories does it bring up? What patterns does it show? What purpose is there in the problem; in the help sought?
3. *What is your goal?* What aim do you have now? What is changing as you talk about your problem and about yourself?
4. *How are you going to do it?* How are you going to commit yourself to the new vision? What practical steps are you going to change?

If we can be there for someone, listen attentively, and be guided by some of the experience above, then we will certainly do no harm and will probably find we have been able to help.

REFERENCES

British Association for Counselling (BAC) (1989) *Code of Ethics and Practice for Counselling Skills*. Rugby: BAC.

British Association for Counselling (BAC) (1995) *Counselling: Definition of Terms in Use* (information sheet no. 1). Rugby: BAC.

British Association for Counselling (BAC) (1996) *Code of Ethics and Practice for Supervisors of Counsellors*. Rugby: BAC.

Brown, D. & Pedder, J. (1979) *Introduction to Psychotherapy: an Outline of Psychodynamic Principles and Practice*. London: Tavistock Publications.

Cunningham, C. & Davis, H. (1985) *Working with Parents: Frameworks for Collaboration*. Milton Keynes: Open University Press.

Ersser, S. (1991) A search for the therapeutic dimensions of nurse–patient interaction. In *Nursing as Therapy*, ed. MacMahon, R. London: Chapman Hall.

Jacobs, M. (1986) *The Presenting Past – an Introduction to Practical Psychodynamic Counselling*. London: Harper and Row.

Kelly, G. (1991) *The Psychology of Personal Constructs*. London: Routledge.

Kfir, N. (1989) *Crisis Intervention Verbatim*. London: Hemisphere Publishing.

Nelson-Jones, R. (1993) *You Can Help! Introducing Life Skills Helping*. London: Cassell.

Page, F. (1984) Gestalt therapy. In *Individual Therapy in Britain*, ed. Dryden, W. London: Harper and Row.

Rogers, C.R. (1951) *Client-centred Therapy*. Boston: Houghton-Mifflin.

Rogers, C. (1961) *On Becoming a Person*. London: Constable.

Savage, J. (1995) *Nursing Intimacy: an Ethnographic Approach to Nurse Patient Interaction*. London: Scutari Press.

Scholes, J. (1996) Therapeutic use of self. *Nursing in Critical Care*, **1(2)**, 60–66.

Spufford, M. (1989) *Celebration*. London: Fount Paperbacks.

Stewart, W. (1979) *Health Service Counselling*. London: Pitman Medical.

Stewart, W. (1997) *An A–Z of Counselling Theory and Practice*, 2nd edn. Cheltenham: Stanley Thornes.

Thorne, B. (1984) Person-centred therapy. In: *Individual Therapy in Britain*, ed. Dryden, W. London: Harper and Row.

Tschudin, V. (1995) *Counselling Skills for Nurses*, 4th edn. London: Baillière Tindall.

Winnicott, D. (1958) *Collected Papers: Through Paediatrics to Psycho-analysis*. London: Tavistock Publications.

Winnicott, D. (1986) *Home is Where We Start From*. London: Penguin.

Wright, B. (1986) *Caring in Crisis – a Handbook of Intervention Skills for Nurses*. Edinburgh: Churchill Livingstone.

FURTHER READING

Altschuler, J. (1997) *Working with Chronic Illness*. London: Macmillan Press.

Bayne, R., Horton, I., Merry, T. & Noyes, E. (1994) *The Counsellor's Handbook: a Practical A–Z Guide to Professional and Clinical Practice*. London: Chapman and Hall.

Bayne, R., Nicholson, P. & Horton, I. (eds) (1998) *Counselling and Communication Skills for Medical and Health Practitioners*. Leicester: BPS Books.

British Association for Counselling – Counselling in Medical Setting Division (1995) *Guidelines for Staff Employed to Counsel in Hospital and Health Care Settings*. Rugby: BAC.

Burnard, P. (1994) *Counselling Skills for Health Professionals*, 2nd edn. London: Chapman and Hall.

Burnard, P. (1992) *Counselling: a Guide to Practice in Nursing*. London: Butterworth Heineman.

Crompton, M. (1992) *Children and Counselling*. London: Edward Arnold.

Davis, H. (1993) *Counselling Parents of Children with Chronic Illness or Disability*. Leicester: BPS Books.

Dryden, W. (ed) (1984) *Individual Therapy in Britain*. London: Harper and Row.

Dryden, W. & Feltham, C. (1992) *Brief Counselling*. Buckingham: Open University Press.

East, P. (1995) *Counselling in Medical Settings*. Buckingham: Open University Press.

Edwards, M. & Davis, H. (1997) *Counselling Children with Chronic Medical Conditions*. Leicester: BPS Books.

Egan, G. (1998) *The Skilled Helper*, 6th edn. Belmont, CA: Brookes/Cole Publishing.

Faulkner, A. (1992) *Effective Interaction with Patients*. Books for Project 2000. Edinburgh: Churchill Livingstone.

Geldard, K. & Geldard, D. (1997) *Counselling Children – a Practical Introduction*. London: Sage.

Inskipp, F. (1996) *Skills Training for Counselling*. London: Cassell.

Jacobs, M. (1985) *Swift to Hear*. London: SPCK.

Kagan, C. & Evans, J. (1995) *Professional Interpersonal Skills for Nurses*. London: Chapman and Hall.

Mellish, V. (1996) Counselling and Support in Intensive Care. *Nursing in Critical Care*, **1(3)**, 116–119.

Noonan, E. (1996) *Counselling Young People*, 2nd edn. London: Tavistock/Routledge.

Rogers, C. (1980) *A Way of Being*. Boston: Houghton Mifflin.

Tschudin, V. (1994) *Counselling: a Primer for Nurses. Workbook and Workshop Guide*. London: Baillière Tindall.

Tschudin, V. (1997) *Counselling for Loss and Bereavement*. London: Baillière Tindall.

Worden, J.W. (1991) *Grief Counselling and Grief Therapy*, 2nd edn. London: Routledge.

Wright, B. (1991) *Sudden Death – Intervention Skills for the Caring Professions*. Edinburgh: Churchill Livingstone.

Organ donation and children

9

INTRODUCTION

Organ donation is probably not a topic of regular discussion. Most people would rather not think about it, either because they hope they will never need to receive a transplanted organ or because they cannot bear to imagine what it would be like to have a close relation in the situation of being a possible donor.

Many children die whilst waiting for a transplant, before a suitable donor organ becomes available. Some may be maintained on dialysis whilst waiting for kidneys, but their quality of life is poor and there is great stress on the family nursing the child and frequently visiting hospitals. Machines cannot maintain a failing heart or liver and these children would have a better chance of a successful transplant if they were to have their operations before their condition became life-threatening.

This chapter explains the procedures and explores the issues for the family and staff when a child is an organ donor. An insight into what is involved will hopefully provide the background information for those who offer support and counselling to the bereaved families afterwards. Relatively few hospitals have experience of working with transplant patients, so it is understandable that most medical and nursing staff would find it difficult to speak with knowledge and confidence about organ donation and transplantation.

A flow chart detailing the stages of organ donation from brain stem death to final funeral arrangements is given in Figure 9.1.

IMPORTANT ISSUES FOR STAFF

Intensive care units, particularly neurosurgical and trauma units, may care for adult patients who become donors, but are generally anxious when the patient is a child. Staff need to be extremely sensitive to the needs of patients and their families, which only

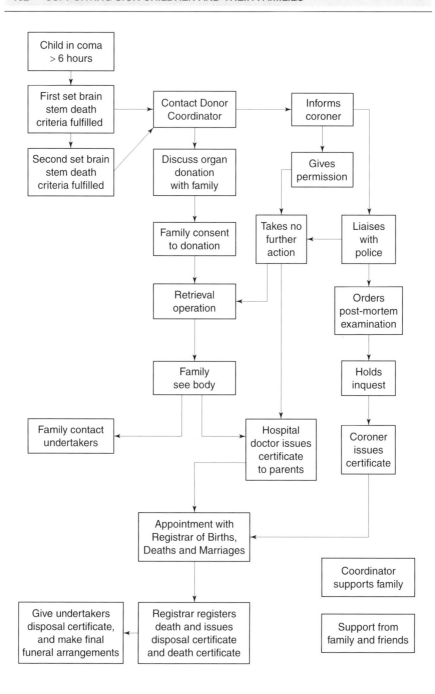

Fig. 9.1 Summary of the procedure of organ donation.

adds to their fears of handling the situation well. Critical care nurses are more likely to recognise a potential donor than any other member of the health care team (Gibson 1995).

This is an area of work where it is particularly important for staff to have thought about their own feelings on the different issues that may arise. If they have not addressed any difficulties for themselves then it will be even harder when faced with patients' relatives, who are looking to them for guidance and support. The issue of organ donation is a difficult one for nurses, but a full understanding of the facts is vital if the nurse is to give guidance and support to relatives (Thomas, 1991). Johnson (1992) argues that some nurses seem unprepared and unable to deal with the emotions of the patient's family and with the ethical and moral issues involved.

Many staff have not thought about the subject enough to carry a donor card themselves; perhaps they should ask themselves why this is. Alternatively, they may have moral or religious objections to donation and transplantation, and sometimes a previous experience has a negative effect on later thinking. If staff do have strong feelings against donation and transplantation, then it is sensible to decide whether they should be working in that area at all, unless they are able to put their own opinions aside for the sake of the family in their care. There are many ways in which staff can be helped to understand this subject.

It is important to let your relatives know how you feel about organ donation and to carry a card. The NHS Organ Donor Register is a computer database of people who wish to register themselves as organ donors; forms for this are freely available through health centres and many public offices. The register is set up by the United Kingdom Transplant Support Service Authority, which is a special health authority of the NHS based near Bristol. They produce several publications, including a booklet of questions and straight answers about transplants (UK Transplant Support Service Authority, 1994).

There is still a shortage of organs available for those on the waiting lists for transplants.

THE ROLE OF THE TRANSPLANT CO-ORDINATORS

The regional transplant coordinators play a large part in promoting awareness and understanding of organ donation. They give talks to groups in towns, villages and schools, and are frequent exhibitors at conferences and public events.

The coordinators arrange study days, workshops and conferences for health professionals. In some areas, a transplant link nurses forum has been established. One of the many benefits from these educational events is the opportunity to think about organ donation and transplantation with other colleagues. This includes learning about brain stem death, approaching relatives, care of donors and also hearing what it is like to wait for an organ and what a successful transplant might mean to a patient.

The donor coordinator responds to a call from an intensive care unit advising of a possible donor by giving advice to the staff and visiting the patient's family to explain about donation. A coordinator is available 24 hours a day and liaises with the donor hospital, UK transplant service and the recipient hospital. The role also includes collecting all the information needed to select a suitable recipient and arranging the retrieval operation. An important duty is to the donor's family, who depend on the coordinator for information and support before, during and after the retrieval operation.

THE CRITERIA FOR ORGAN DONATION

Nurses in intensive care units need to understand which patients could be suitable organ donors; one of a series of leaflets for health care professionals written by the UK Transplant Coordinators' Association (undated) explains:

The potential organ donor is a patient in whom brain stem death has been confirmed and who is being maintained on a ventilator. Common pathologies resulting in brain stem death include:
- cerebral trauma
- intracranial haemorrhage
- anoxic brain damage, e.g. following cardiac or respiratory arrest, smoke inhalation or drowning
- primary brain tumour.

The following factors would exclude a patient from becoming a donor:
- age more than 75 years. There is no lower age limit
- malignant disease except primary brain tumour
- major systemic sepsis
- positive hepatitis B surface antigen test
- positive HIV antibody test.

CARING FOR THE FAMILIES OF POTENTIAL ORGAN DONORS

When we consider the group of patients who could be donors, we should recognise that most of the medical conditions leading to brain stem death are a result of a sudden severe illness or trauma. This means that family members are likely to be numb from the shock and will hardly be able to believe what is happening; it will not yet seem real. Careful timing of the giving of information and the request for decisions is therefore extremely important.

Let us consider a child admitted to intensive care with major head injuries, a low Glasgow Coma Score and unresponsive pupils. The prognosis on arrival would be poor but not hopeless at this stage. The parents will need to be with their child and to be kept informed of the condition and changes as they happen. They will need to feel they can trust those caring for their child, and will feel helpless and desperate.

If the parents are to understand and accept brain stem death in their child, they must have understood the stages leading up to that; building on what they know is helpful. Honesty helps with developing trust, so be honest right from the start with a clear assessment of the child's condition and the treatment plan.

Explanations of regular neurological observations, monitoring, drugs and scans will help in the building of the full picture that allows the parents to see for themselves the hopeless situation. If someone can be alongside the parents at these stages – a nurse, doctor, counsellor or chaplain – to help them express their feelings and thoughts, it is a way of checking that they have understood what has been said and to correct any misunderstandings. Giving time is very supportive even if there are periods when not much is said. There must be times for the parents to be together on their own, to share their fears and concerns.

BRAIN STEM DEATH

Helping the family to understand

Brain stem death is not easy for medically educated personnel to comprehend at first, so great care must be taken to ensure that the parents understand there is no hope of recovery. It must be incredibly hard to believe your child is dead when warm and pink with a chest going up and down as in breathing. This demonstrates the importance of ensuring at an early stage that the family understands that a ventilator is a machine that breathes for you and not, as it is frequently called, a 'life support machine'. They have to trust the professionals involved when they are told that their child's brain is dead, and some families need to see this for themselves. It should be made clear to the family members that they are not expected to witness the tests;

for some it would be more than they could bear at this time.

It is advisable for the medical consultant carrying out the tests to agree to a family member being present if he or she so wishes. Some doctors find it distressing to face the parents while doing the tests and this should be respected and another doctor asked to carry them out. It is courteous and caring if the doctor is introduced to the parent and explains what is to be done. Someone should be available to sit down with them, a short distance from the bed, and talk through what is happening. This also allows time for parents to talk and to express their feelings. It may become too hard to bear and they could faint or need helping out of the room. It is possible that a grandparent or an aunt or uncle will choose to be present instead of the parents.

Brain stem death tests

- The patient must have been in deep coma for at least 6 hours before considering brain stem death tests.
- The tests must be performed twice, by two experienced doctors, either two consultants or one consultant and a senior registrar. One of them must not have been involved in the patient's care and neither should be involved in transplantation.
- There is no set time lapse between the two sets of tests; it may be extended to allow the family to discuss and reach a decision on donation.
- The confirmed time of death is when the second set of criteria have been fulfilled. This point should be explained to the family to avoid further confusion later (see Case Study 9.1).

Before brain stem death can be diagnosed, it must be established that:

- the patient is unresponsive, on a ventilator
- there is a clear cause of coma due to irremediable structural brain damage

---

CASE STUDY 9.1 *Time of death in cases of brain stem death*

Sandra prefers to think that her son died at their home; she was probably right, as he arrested and was resuscitated at home by the paramedical team. The following day, in the paediatric intensive care unit, he fulfilled brain stem death criteria and that became the confirmed time of death. Both his parents were comfortable with the thought that the child died at home, but the official date was the following day.

- there is no potential for reversible apnoeic coma conditions; these include
  — drug effects on the central nervous system
  — shock and hypotension from recent circulatory arrest
  — metabolic and endocrine disorders
  — primary hypothermia.

Absence of the brain stem reflexes indicates loss of brain stem function, and the criteria for establishing this are presented in Box 9.1; alongside these criteria are the explanations that might be given to parents.

Box 9.1 Criteria for establishing absence of brain stem reflexes	
Medical terminology	Lay terminology (for parents and family)
No pupillary response to light	No change in pupil size
No corneal reflex	No blinking
No vestibular-occular reflex	No eye movement
No motor responses within the cranial nerve distribution area to painful stimulation	No grimace
No gag reflex after tracheal stimulation	No gag or cough
Apnoea test following strict criteria	No attempt to breathe

Telling the family that brain stem death has been established

When the brain stem death criteria have been fulfilled, the result has to be given to the family. Most parents decide not to be present and are content with an explanation of what the tests are – simple tests carried out at the bedside to establish that there is no nerve response from the brain and that the patient cannot make any attempt to breathe.

A quiet room away from the clinical area should be available for talking to the family, with enough seats for everyone and tissues at hand. If the family members have been well prepared for the expected outcome of the testing, then it will merely confirm what they suspected but hoped would not be true. The doctor, who they should have already met, could say: 'We have completed the special tests on Simon, and I'm afraid it is as we thought. They have proved that his brain is dead. I am so sorry.' The relatives who have been at the bedside may nod through their tears and say they knew what they would be told and that they felt the person was not there any more.

The parents may need to telephone other relatives, such as their parents, if they are not present, and it is helpful if they can use a telephone in a private place. If they are too distressed to dial the numbers correctly or to speak to the relatives themselves, they may appreciate a member of staff doing this for them. I hope this emphasises the value of having someone from the team available for the family at all stages. The distressed family needs back-up explanations from someone who heard what the doctor said when they could not take it all in, who can make useful suggestions, be a sounding board, and guide them through the useful situation. This is a hard time for the staff, but I know how much the family members need and appreciate their support, and how gratefully they will remember the kindness afterwards.

Brothers and sisters need not be excluded from the discussions and decisions. Older children are often able to understand that the brain is the nerve centre of the body and liken it to a programmed computer – if the brain is not working then the body cannot work as it does not receive or give any messages. I have seen a 12-year-old listen very carefully while a consultant showed him scans and carefully and simply explained the condition of his brother's brain and why it could not recover. It helped him to feel valued and part of what was happening.

After the first set of criteria has been fulfilled, the family need to be guided very carefully and sensitively through the following hours. The doctor will explain that a colleague has to repeat the same tests and will indicate a time for this to take place. If the subject of organ donation has not been discussed already then now is the time to raise it, preferably by someone whom the family know and trust.

If the parents do not think of donation during quiet times on their own or when talking with relatives, they may raise the subject at the bedside and ask the nurse about it. This highlights the importance of nurses being familiar with the facts, as it would be appropriate in this instance for the nurse to continue with the discussion and ask the correct professionals to take their part in the procedure.

Organ donation is sometimes discussed with the family before brain stem death has been established, if relatives have chosen to do this, but more often the subject is raised after the first of the two sets of tests.

RAISING THE QUESTION OF ORGAN DONATION

It is often in quiet periods that parents raise the subject of organ donation. If they have come to accept that their child is going to die, they may say something like: 'If nothing more can be done to help our child, is there any way he can help someone else?' This is a good cue to continue with: 'Perhaps you have been thinking that he might be an organ donor'; 'I wonder if you have ever thought about organ donation'; or 'Do you know if he carried a donor card?'

If the parents do not raise the subject, and there is no reason to expect them to, then a member of the medical or nursing staff or the transplant co-ordinator would do so. Whoever does broach the subject must be sure of the facts and confident with the task. Many medical and nursing staff understandably find it difficult to ask the family members if they would like to donate their loved one's organs for transplantation (Morgan, 1995) so it is important that the person making the request has the trust and confidence of the family.

The manner of death precipitating the possibility of organ donation is invariably sudden and tragic, evoking many and varied emotions for both family and medical and nursing staff; such emotions can impede communication (Franklin, Crombie & Nicholls, 1996).

The immediate responses of parents will cover all the possibilities: some will be firmly in favour, others firmly against, while most will be uncertain. It is important to understand that these immediate responses may not be final decisions; many parents change their view after they have had time to think and talk about what is involved.

When many members of a family are involved in making the decisions, it may take longer to reach agreement. It is often the older generation who have not thought about organ transplantation before and they may say they do not agree with it instead of admitting they do not understand it. If someone, perhaps a nurse, doctor or transplant coordinator, is able to spend time helping them to understand what is involved, and explaining how other children could benefit, they may find the idea more acceptable. An 80-year-old grandmother I came across found the idea hard to accept, but was helped in this by the memory that her grandchild had always been kind and wanting to help other people, and that his parents were blood donors. It may be the child's parents or legal guardians who sign the consent form for organ donation, but it is always easier to make the decision, and to live comfortably with it afterwards, if all the family are in agreement.

Considering issues of religion

Advice or reassurance from a minister of religion may be helpful in the discussion. Individual personal wishes must be respected, but the Christian churches do not have ethical objections to organ donation and transplantation. Hindus, Sikhs and Buddhists generally have no objections and Jewish law states that organs should not be removed until complete cessation of all spontaneous life functions. Islamic law requires Muslims to be buried as soon as possible after death so organ donation may be refused. Jehovah's Witnesses are advised that organ donation and receiving organs are personal decisions.

Children know about organ donation

Many children have discussed organ donation at school and perhaps heard a transplant coordinator speak, or they may have heard about somebody who had a transplant. I have heard young people refer to the use of organs when someone dies as merely recycling!

Refusal to allow donation

When a request is refused it may be worth asking if there are any questions parents would like to ask, as a means of ensuring that the refusal is final; otherwise their wishes must be respected. It would seem better to ask about donation and be refused rather than be afraid to ask and find out later that the family would have liked to donate but did not think of it themselves until it was too late. It may be worth saying this to relatives.

BODY, the British Organ Donor Society, have produced two excellent booklets for families (BODY, 1991, 1993). They are easy to understand and address many of the issues facing the families. They can prove very helpful when making the decision to allow donation.

Which organs can be used?

Parents will want to know which organs can be used, and are often surprised to hear how many recipients there might be. They have probably thought of kidneys, but did not know they could go to two different people. If the child does not have damage to any organs then it may be possible to donate heart and lungs, liver and corneas as well as kidneys. In some regions, it is possible to save bone and skin from older children, to be used for grafting. A few specialised centres may have children waiting for small bowel and/or pancreas transplants. If certain organs are not suitable for donation then it is important to explain this to the parents; otherwise they could misunderstand and wonder why their child was not good enough. It is not uncommon for a parent to be specific about which organs to donate. One father asked me which 'bits' could be used, so I explained which were the possible organs. As I mentioned the heart, his wife burst out crying, saying she could not bear to give his heart. She felt bad for saying so and did not know why she felt so strongly, but was quite definite, so they agreed willingly to donate the kidneys and liver, but not the heart.

WHEN ORGAN DONATION HAS BEEN AGREED

It is usual for the transplant coordinator to become involved at this stage, if not before, and he or she will explain what happens and answer questions. A multi-organ donor must be a 'beating heart donor', which means that the person must go to theatre for the retrieval operation while still on the ventilator, in order to keep the organs fully perfused. This has proved to be a difficulty for a few parents who desperately want to be holding their child as the heart stops. They want to feel that the child died in their arms. This would mean that the heart, lungs or liver could not be used. If the parents remain firm on this point, and yet would still like to donate something, then it is usually possible to give kidneys if the retrieval can be arranged within 45 minutes of the death. Corneas and heart valves may be taken after death or at post-mortem examination.

Reassurance must be given that the child will be treated with respect throughout the procedure and that the abdomen will be stitched after the operation. Parents like to know that the transplant coordinator or a nurse will stay with the child in the theatre and will bring the child back afterwards.

The confirmed time of death

The confirmed time of death is when the second set of brain stem death criteria have been fulfilled, so if a formal identification must be made after death then it may be done at this point. If the coroner is involved and there is to be a postmortem examination and possible inquest then a police officer must witness a relative making the identification. This sounds very formal and frightening for distressed parents, but it is often better for them to do this at the bedside than to make a formal visit to the hospital chapel of rest later on. The police officer will gently ask the parents if this is their child and say the name. When they agree, the statement is signed and the police go away to complete their paperwork for the coroner's officer. The coordinator will inform the coroner of a possible donor, giving the medical history, as permission is needed if there is to be a coroner's postmortem examination and inquest.

Caring for the family while waiting for the retrieval operation

After the family have agreed to organ donation, care of the patient as well as the family members will continue. The role of the nurse changes, from striving positively for the benefit of the child, to careful preservation of a body in the best condition for donation. This is not easy for nurses, who will be sad at the loss of a young life despite their best efforts and distressed from being alongside the family through their anxieties and deep emotions. It is a continuation of care, and for relatives it becomes desperately important because they hold onto the hope that something positive will come out of this terrible tragedy.

Some parents choose to stay beside their child, taking a real interest in the details of preparing for donation. Once brain stem death has been established, there is a risk that the patient may become haemodynamically unstable and unsuitable as a donor, so the transplant coordinator must not delay in making the many arrangements leading up to a theatre time for the retrieval operation. It may be helpful to explain to the parents the importance of frequent checking of blood gases, electrolytes, fluid balance, as well as blood tests for hepatitis B and C and HIV.

Whilst all the necessary care is continuing at the bedside, it must be remembered that for the parents, these are the last precious few hours with their child. Parents will want to ensure that every detail has been taken care of, including all aspects of their child's appearance. Some may prefer nurses to do this, but most families like to join in and help with, for example, washing and brushing hair. A parent may want to lie on the bed too, play quiet music or read to the child; it is a tranquil and dignified time. It may be supportive to sit quietly beside the parents at regular intervals, to offer tea or coffee and allow time for them to talk about how they are feeling. They often ask what they have to do next, and make comments about their early plans for the funeral, which cans make them feel guilty as the child is still with them. This is natural and shows that they are accepting the reality of the situation. It also gives them something to think about, to take their thoughts beyond the present moments, and so may be their way of coping with what is happening. Whatever their thoughts, it does seem important to help them to make the last hours with their child a peaceful memory.

THE RETRIEVAL OPERATION

When the anaesthetist and theatre assistants arrive, the portable ventilator, monitors and pumps are connected and the bed is moved out of the unit to the theatre. The nurse who had been looking after the child will probably go with them, and may even choose to go into theatre. There is something important about seeing a special task through to the end, and there is perhaps an added sense of responsibility on behalf of the parents. It certainly seems to give comfort to know that the nurse will be with the child. The parents may follow them out through the doors, but it is advisable for someone to accompany them to a quiet place to allow them to cry, talk and just be together alone.

The retrieval usually takes at least 4 or 5 hours, and often longer, depending on how many surgical teams are involved. The family need to know this and should be offered guidance in planning what to do during this time. Some parents decide to stay at the hospital, while others prefer to go home and return later or the next day if it is during the evening. Relatives who stay at the hospital may like to spend the time privately in a quiet place, or perhaps visit the hospital chapel. They may feel able to eat some food 'to keep up their strength' or possibly only be able to drink and eat very little. Frequent offers of tea and coffee are important to prevent dehydration in warm surroundings and these may be the only form of energy being taken when so much energy is being used up in this highly stressful situation. The parents may be too physically exhausted to drive home, or have no transport, so it would be sensible to offer them somewhere to lie down and try to sleep.

The need to keep in touch continues, whether the parents stay at the hospital or go home. They know that there is nothing more they can do for their child but there is a strong sense of caring, responsibility and interest in the organ donation.

SEEING THE BODY AFTERWARDS

During the retrieval operation, preparations can be started for the family to see the child's body after completion. Thought must be given as to where this should take place. If there is no special quiet room, then a side room on the unit or ward could be made available, or a treatment or preparation room could be put out of general use temporarily. It is appropriate for the child to be returned to a room close to that in which care was provided prior to the retrieval operation as the area of the hospital and the staff will be familiar. The family may, however, prefer to see the child's body in a different place, as this can help them to feel their child has moved on and that they are in the next stage. The hospital chapel of rest could be suitable. The aim is to provide a peaceful environment for the family to be together and say goodbye; it is perhaps also to keep an earlier promise that the child would be brought back to them after the operation.

If the room is normally a clinical area, then try to remove or cover some equipment. Use soft, low lights, a cot or bed with children's bed linen and perhaps some flowers at the side to help soften the atmosphere. Dress the child in whatever clothes the parents choose, or find something suitable on the ward. The abdominal wound will be closed and all skin cleaned perfectly. Padding will be used to restore normal shape to the eyes and the eyelids will be stitched down. It helps to be prepared for the shock of seeing the white skin colour, due to the loss of blood. Pay particular attention to cleaning the nails as the family will probably hold the hands, and brush the hair, which they may stroke. Do not forget to put the favourite soft toy in the bed. The nurse or nurses who have cared for this child may like to attend to these details; it is a way for them to complete their tasks in caring for the child and family and for them personally to say goodbye. The transplant coordinator may also like to help. The parents and siblings may choose to add a final personal touch of their own, such as laying a flower, special toy or message.

The family may not stay to see the child or want to come back at that time, in which case the body will be taken to the mortuary. Arrangements should be made for them to visit the next day, perhaps in the chapel of rest, after checking the time of the post-mortem examination with the mortuary staff.

Some parents and families may think they would rather not see the child's body and just 'remember him as he was'. This is understandable at a time of great distress, but it must be stressed that in the days, weeks and even months ahead, the parents may have real problems in their grieving if they have not been able to see their child dead and had an opportunity to say goodbye. It has been known for parents to believe that their child is not dead, but still at the hospital. Staff may need to give much patient encouragement and support to enable them to acknowledge the awful reality.

LEAVING THE HOSPITAL

When the family leave the hospital, make sure they have telephone numbers to ring if they have any questions or problems. Sometimes they may like to ring just to speak to someone who was there with them and who knows what has happened without having to be told. For this reason, the hospital staff become special to them, which makes it even more important to care for them well. Check that the family has transport home, or that someone is fit to drive.

The transplant coordinator will thank the family for their generous gift and promise to write to them with information about recipients of the organs. They do not give personal details, but will tell them which organs were used, e.g. a 26-year-old mother received one kidney, a 14-year-old boy the other.

THANKING THOSE WHO HELPED

It is appreciated if the transplant coordinator writes to the medical and nursing staff who were involved with the donor to thank them for their help and cooperation. This would include the intensive care unit staff and the theatre staff. They should be informed of the outcome of the retrieval, which helps to complete the care and attention given to the family, and values their role in the team. It may go some way towards addressing a possible sense of frustration at the failure of treatment to save the child's life.

SUPPORTING THE STAFF

The intensity and sensitivity of this area of work are such that staff should be free to express choice over caring for a patient with brain stem death. There must be adequate time for short breaks away from the bedside for refreshment, and frequent contact with colleagues checking they remain comfortable in the situation. It can be very supportive to share feelings with another team member who takes the time to listen, preferably a colleague who has been through this experience before and so can listen with empathy.

BEREAVEMENT SUPPORT OF A DONOR'S FAMILY

The letter from the coordinator to the family becomes a very precious legacy of a tragic death. It may be the only positive thing to come from it and so it is important to send a carefully written letter that the family will treasure. I know parents who carry this letter around in their wallets and some who have displayed it at the funeral.

Some parents have felt that donating organs has helped them in their grief and want to tell other people what they have done. A number of families will tell their story to a local newspaper, especially if the death has become public knowledge, such as following a road traffic accident. This publicity helps to increase awareness of the need for organ donation by encouraging other people to think about it and to carry donor cards.

Bereaved parents often dream about their dead child, especially during the first few weeks after the death, and for most parents this is quite natural and pleasant. I have heard parents describe some weird dreams after their child was an organ donor, which have left them feeling rather unsettled. The unpleasant thoughts they remember often have to do with issues of dismemberment of the child's body.

One mother described a feeling of being haunted by her decision to allow her child to be 'cut up'. Fortunately these dreams did not last for long, and it was helpful for the parents to talk about them to a counsellor who allowed the frightening feelings to be expressed. It was reassuring to hear that other parents had experienced similar dreams, and to make sense out of them. Parents often experience some guilt that they have allowed their child to be 'used' and a strange realisation that parts of their child, who is dead, are in other people who are alive. These unnerving thoughts and feelings are part of the expected pattern of grief – the guilt, searching for reasons for the death of their child, and anger at the loss.

Parents often benefit from sharing their feelings with other donor families and from the discovery that their thoughts and reactions are not unexpected in their situation. Most parents have found that, with patient support and time to talk, they are able to move on in their grieving. They are able to know that they have done something very special for someone unknown to them and they take comfort from this. The British Organ Donor Society (BODY) holds a service of remembrance each year and has arranged the planting of an avenue of trees in the grounds of Wimpole Hall* in Cambridgeshire. Each tree is planted by a family in memory of someone who died and was an organ donor, or by a grateful recipient.

Most transplant coordinators offer to keep in touch with families for a while after the death, and some visit them at home. This keeps a link with the hospital and gives parents the opportunity to return to talk with the doctors and nurses and to ask questions. It is helpful to give families the contact telephone numbers for CRUSE bereavement care, Compassionate Friends, the British Organ Donor Society and any local group for bereaved parents.

The loss of a child is always hard to bear, and for these families there are extra issues to work through. It is so important for them to feel supported and to know where to go for help in the difficult weeks and months ahead.

CONCLUSION

This chapter has described procedures leading up to a child becoming an organ donor and considered some of the issues around that decision. Detailed information has been given in order to prepare health professionals with facts they might not have the opportunity of learning until they are faced with caring for a potential child organ donor and a family who look to them for support. It may be appropriate to read the following chapter as well, as this considers support for families of children who receive transplanted organs.

The death of a child, especially when it is sudden or the result of a tragic accident, is never going to be easy for the family or the staff caring for them. The question of donating organs may be thought to complicate matters, but many grieving families take some comfort from knowing they gave hope to others (see also Chs 14 and 15).

---

*Wimpole Hall, Arrington, Royston SG8 0BW, is on A603, 8 miles SW of Cambridge. The house, farm and park belong to the National Trust and are open to the public. The park is open free every day.

REFERENCES

BODY (1991) The gift of life – an introduction to organ and tissue transplantation. Balsham, Cambridge: British Organ Donor Society.

BODY (1993) The gift of life 2 – a handbook for donor families. Balsham, Cambridge: British Organ Donor Society.

Franklin, P., Crombie, A. & Nicholls, J. (1996) Organ donation – discussing the option with the family. *Care of the Critically Ill*, **12(3)**, 95–96.

Gibson, V. (1995) Nurses' experiences of organ donation. *Care of the Critically Ill*, **11(5)**, 176.

Johnson, C. (1992) The nurse's role in organ donation from a brainstem dead patient: management of the family. *Intensive and Critical Care Nursing*, **8**, 140–148.

Morgan, V. (1995) Brain stem death testing and consent for cadaveric organ donation. *Care of the Critically Ill*, **11(1)**, 20–22.

Thomas, S. (1991) The gift of life. *Nursing Times*, **87(37)**, 28–31.

UK Transplant Co-ordinators Association. *Organ Donation and Transplantation; Religious and Cultural Issues; Brain Stem Death; Why Carry the Card?* London: HMSO. (Information leaflets for healthcare professionals.)

UK Transplant Support Service Authority (1994) *Questions and Straight Answers about Transplants.* Bristol: UKTSSA. (Available from UKTSSA, Fox Den Road, Stoke Gifford, Bristol BS12 6RR.)

FURTHER READING

Department of Health and Social Security (1983) *Cadaveric Organs for Transplantation, a Code of Practice including the Diagnosis of Brain Stem Death.* London: HMSO.

Pallis, C. (1983) *ABC of Brain Stem Death.* London: BMJ.

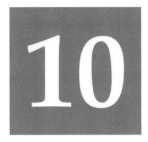

Organ transplantation for children

INTRODUCTION

It may seem a little surprising to include a chapter on organ transplantation, considering how few children receive transplanted organs or tissue, but it is because not many professionals have experience in this highly specialised field that I feel it is important to think about it in this book. Most general practitioners, health visitors, school nurses, outpatient clinic staff and school teachers will not meet a child who has had a transplant in their whole career. Those who do have to care for these children have a great deal to learn about the relevant procedures and the emotional as well as the physical needs of the child and family.

I hope this chapter goes some way towards helping them to understand what the family has to endure and experience, and thus to enable them to be supportive. The whole process of transplantation can cause intense psychological distress and considerable social disruption for the patient and family (Froment, 1992).

Early attempts at transplanting organs from one human to another did not have successful long-term outcomes because of the problems of rejection. With the introduction of new anti-rejection drugs in the late 1970s, the results improved, as they continue so to do with more drugs available. Transplantation is now the treatment of choice for many children with failing organs – livers, kidneys, hearts and lungs. Bone marrow transplants are increasing and skin grafts, corneal grafts and small bowel transplants are being performed for children.

The process of organ transplantation for a child has a profound impact on the whole family; parents are faced with a number of psychosocial stresses many of which are unique in a paediatric hospital setting (Gold *et al.*, 1986). Newspapers use headings such as 'liver swap girl' as if the process was as easy as replacing a spare part in a car, with little or no knowledge of the actual facts. When assessing the success of transplantation, it is imperative that equal weighting is given to both objective and subjective data so that the full story can be told (Maynard, 1993). Time spent with the child, parents and siblings to help them explore their own understanding and feelings is an essential part of the family care.

THE CHILD BEING CONSIDERED FOR TRANSPLANTATION

Children who come for transplantation have different presentations and medical histories, depending on the diagnosis and organ concerned, the length of illness and state of health or severity of symptoms. For all of them, the chance of a transplant may be the only possibility of an improved quality of life; for most, it is the only chance of a future life.

Liver transplants

The child may have been born with a condition involving the liver, such as biliary atresia when the bile ducts are insufficient or absent. If this condition is not diagnosed and treated early enough (when only a few weeks old), the liver function tests will become abnormal and the baby will not thrive because of a failing liver.

It is devastating for parents to learn that their baby, whom they thought was normal and healthy at birth, has a life-threatening condition. Biliary atresia is not genetically inherited and there is no prenatal diagnosis, so it is a shock, even though they may have been worried that the baby was jaundiced. It is hard to convince parents that there was nothing they could have done to prevent this, and they often feel guilty.

Other liver conditions may not lead to deterioration so early and the child may enjoy a good life for some years before a transplant is considered. Children of school age may suffer cruel teasing about their yellow skin colour or for not having the stamina to take part in sport. Some cannot walk up stairs or for any distance, due to arthropathy or rickets. Girls have problems finding trendy clothes to fit over a large abdomen. These factors may help older children to have a positive approach to the operation and recovery afterwards.

Kidney transplants

A child with chronic renal failure may be on regular dialysis for some time before being able to have a kidney transplant. During this time, the general health and development of the child and the quality of life for the whole family are likely to deteriorate. In a study carried out by Reynolds *et al.*(1991), most parents rated their child's physical health as considerably improved after transplantation, and noted improvements in the child's behaviour and in the quality of family life.

Children with cystic fibrosis

Some children with cystic fibrosis develop signs of liver failure and enjoy real benefit from a liver transplant. Some older children, usually teenagers or young adults, have lung or heart-and-lung transplants. They continue to have cystic fibrosis, but if the operation is successful they have much improved health. These young people should have every opportunity to ask their own questions and be part of the discussions so that they can make informed decisions about their future treatment.

Heart transplants

Children waiting for heart transplants may have congenital heart disease, a chronic heart condition or a failing heart because of an acute illness, such as a viral infection, that has affected the heart muscle. There is a high mortality during this waiting period; there are also problems of donor–recipient size constraints with children, and sometimes the child may become too sick for the operation.

Small bowel transplants

Relatively few small bowel grafts have been performed on children in Britain, but in the future this procedure could provide hope for children with severe bowel problems, e.g. those born with an abnormally developed small bowel or those who have suffered chronic inflammatory bowel disease. In these cases, intravenous feeding of total parental nutrition may be the only means of giving the child any nourishment, and in time the liver may become damaged, necessitating a liver and small bowel graft. Relying on larger veins for giving intravenous nutrition and medication may in time lead to line infections and difficulties with central venous access.

Bone marrow transplants

Some children with malignant blood disorders, most commonly leukaemia, thalassaemia and immunodeficiency, may be offered bone marrow transplants by the haematology and oncology specialist treatment centres. Bone marrow is given either by donors unknown to the family but whose marrow is compatible with the child, or by a relative, often a compatible sibling.

All of the children being considered for any transplantation are chronically and eventually terminally sick. The majority have been unwell for months or years, but some suffer sudden damage to an organ, usually from an infection (e.g. virus), accident (e.g. lacerated or crushed) or drugs (e.g. paracetamol, chemotherapy), and require emergency transplantation.

Frequent spells in hospital and regular visits for investigations and reviews, in addition to managing a poorly nourished and possibly jaundiced or cyanosed child, are not conducive to a good family life. Siblings may resent the sick child needing so much of the parents' attention and their absence when visiting the hospital.

Mothers have described their loneliness in coping with such a situation; they will have had to learn a great deal themselves in order to understand the child's problems. They give numerous medicines, including perhaps intravenous antibiotics at home, physiotherapy, special diets and perhaps nasogastric feeds. Some have found it impossible to explain everything to grandparents and other relations who could not understand, and welcomed support and companionship from other parents. Caring for the sick child is tiring and stressful and contributes to many broken relationships.

MORAL AND ETHICAL CONSIDERATIONS

Transplantation in children raises considerable moral and ethical issues for the medical and surgical teams and the family. The responsibility for making decisions on a child's behalf must be taken seriously, and the welfare of the child must be paramount (The Children Act, 1989).

The parents may be desperate to allow anything to try to save the child's life and cannot bear to think beyond that. A transplant is never going to provide a magic total cure, as the child will always need medication and the possibility of further treatment and surgery. It is a way of trading one disease for another (Gold *et al.*, 1986) in the hope that the new one is better.

It is perhaps this hope that makes parents go on seeking more and more treatment for their child against all reasonable odds of its success. It is perhaps also their strong sense of responsibility – they are not able, or will not give themselves permission, to let go.

The four basic moral principles advocated by Beauchamp and Childress (1994) are helpful in offering guidance.

1. Respect for people's autonomy or self-determination

As health professionals for these children and their families, we must remember only to impose on them treatments to which we ourselves would consent. This highlights the importance of enabling children to understand procedures as well as their age allows. They must be given honest, accurate information, in language that can be understood. More detail can be given as the child gets older and needs (and wants) to know more. They have a continuing need to make sense of what happened; they have to live with the consequences of adults' decisions made on their behalf. A teenager once asked why his old liver could not have been fixed and why he had to have someone else's (Cook, 1996). He was only 7 years old when he had his transplant operation and information given to him then was no longer sufficient; we must therefore give truthful facts on which to build at a later stage.

We must also consider here the autonomy of a living donor. Is the donor who is emotionally involved with the potential recipient objective enough to make a free decision to take the risks involved in donating an organ to the loved one, or is that person the victim of emotional blackmail (Gillon, 1996)? The potential donor may be too frightened of what others will think if consent is not given with enthusiasm.

It is easy to understand how a parent can expect a sibling to donate marrow. If there is not a compatible sibling, parents have been known to have another baby in the hope that this baby's marrow will be compatible. But is it fair for the baby to be brought up as the saviour of, or replacement for, the sick child?

It is possible in a few situations for a parent to donate a part of their liver to be grafted into the child, where it will regenerate to the right size. Sometimes a relative will donate a kidney. Sufficient time must be given for assessing risks, expressing fears and good psychological support.

2. Non-maleficence or the obligation not to harm

When considering children who would benefit from a successful transplant, most people would recognise that certain risks have to be taken, such as the risks involved in general anaesthesia and major surgery and the possible complications. Since the parents are in the sad situation of knowing that their child will not survive without a transplant, they sometimes comment that there is no harm in trying and nothing to lose in giving the child a chance.

If a living donor is involved, then every care must be taken to ensure that no harm befalls him. Siblings who donate bone marrow must be protected from any psychological trauma – have they consented freely? Will they think it is their fault if the child dies, or that it was their marrow that killed them?

3. Beneficence or the obligation to benefit

The aim of transplantation is for the child to benefit. It is not always easy to see how a donor might benefit, but it can be very satisfying for siblings to feel they have been able to help their brother or sister or for a parent to undergo a donor operation in order to help a child.

We must also consider the possibility that, in cases where the risks are high and the chances of success low, treatment may not be in the child's best interest – it may even be considered abusive. On the other hand, we should not be frightened of trying new procedures – after all, it is worth remembering that some brave surgeon performed the first appendicectomy, and this is now a fairly routine operation.

It is also important to bear in mind, when considering transplantation, that individuals cope differently with the same treatment, and individual parents cope differently with the stresses of their child having to undergo such a difficult and complicated procedure.

4. Justice – the obligation to treat competing claims fairly

The demands on the National Health Service are great and there will always be discussions about high-cost treatment for the few as against lower-cost procedures for the many. Transplants are expensive procedures in terms of money, skills and facilities. There has to be a responsible approach to the use of these resources, treating people in relation to their needs. The parents need reassurance that their child is being treated fairly during the wait for transplant, and that other children 'in competition' for a similar sized organ have not been given priority unless they were more sick. Balancing the pursuit of the good of one individual with that of the common good of all is probably the most important ethical issue in nursing today (Castledine, 1993).

When there are difficulties in deciding what is right for a child, it may be best to take the matter to the courts to decide. Parents do not always have the final say on whether a child has a particular treatment or not, and they may not be in agreement with the medical and surgical opinions. A judge can consider the best interests of the child, and the court can give consent for treatment if necessary.

ASSESSMENT FOR TRANSPLANTATION

Hospitals offering transplants usually have an assessment programme lasting a few days or a week or more. It is important to allow the time for the family to meet all members of the specialist team, especially if they have not met before. There are relatively few centres offering transplants to children, so most families are a long way from home and are unfamiliar with the hospital. They are probably well known at their local centre and may need time to develop trust in the new team.

A family should not be assessed unless transplantation has been discussed at the referral centre, and therefore the problem of ignorance on the part of the family or child should not arise (Warner, 1991). Families need to understand that they are being referred to the specialist centre to explore the possibility of a transplant for their child. Some parents have arrived with a misunderstanding that the transplant would actually take place that week.

The assessment programme may vary but will include:

- confirmation of the diagnosis
- assessment of the child's general state of health and development
- assessment of the involvement of, or damage to, other organs
- assessment by anaesthetist
- assessment by surgeons
- discussions with parents – possible risks, problems, explanation of procedure
- discussion with transplant co-ordinator
- psychosocial issues – time to explore family problems, siblings, employers, support for the family
- preparation for the child as appropriate to age
- visit to intensive care unit and explanation of equipment and postoperative care.

All of these important parts of the assessment will bring particular anxieties for the family, and after a busy week they may feel quite weary and confused. It is important to have a concluding discussion, with every team member in agreement; this united approach is supportive as it suggests confidence rather than confusion.

Time for feelings and emotions

After the results of the tests have been discussed with the parents, it is beneficial to offer some time in a quiet place to reflect on what they have been told, what they understand and what they feel about it. This can be an emotional time as they realise the enormity of the procedures ahead. They will have mixed feelings – the relief that hope of a better life is being offered to their child and numerous fears about the unknown path ahead.

Parents usually say they have no choice but to agree to a transplant as they know the poor prognosis without it. Even if the surgery is not successful, they will have given the child a chance – in one mother's words: 'He would have died without it, so if he dies after the operation at least we gave him the chance'. Hard facts must be discussed – the risks of surgery, long anaesthetic, complications including bleeding, infection, blocking of blood vessels, rejection and a lifetime of taking immunosuppressive drugs. The long-term future and quality of life may remain uncertain, so they should be helped towards realistic expectations.

Warner (1991) is convinced that only the most psychologically robust families who fulfil appropriate criteria should be referred for transplant. This reinforces the importance of assessing the psychosocial alongside the medical issues, and establishing a trusting relationship between the team and the family. The family needs to be well prepared, realistically, for what they can expect to face, how they might feel and what they will be able to do to help themselves, with the support of the team.

The responsibility of parents in making decisions on the child's behalf is enormous. Protective adults who want to spare children the possibility of making harmful decisions, with the ensuing blame and guilt, themselves risk making harmful decisions and being blamed for it by the child at a later date (Alderson, 1993). I know a teenager who still blames his mother for allowing a transplant to be carried out several years ago, even though he has been in good health since.

Thinking about the donor

Receiving a donor organ means that someone will die before the transplant can happen. For some people this is an enormous burden of guilt, while others are able to rationalise it by thinking the person was dying anyway. Parents often find it too painful to think that another family will be grieving for a child while they are given hope. It is often during the assessment discussions that parents start to feel upset by this sensitive issue. It may be helpful for a family to know that they can write anonymously to the donor's family; they may need to know that they will be able to say thank you for the special gift.

The importance of trust

The parents need to be able to trust the medical and nursing staff at all stages, so honesty is vital in building and maintaining trust from the start. A study of coping strategies in parents of children receiving liver transplants (Noble-Jamieson et al., 1996) concluded that parents cope best by having trust in the medical team, by being realistic and by accepting the situation. Giving full information at all stages, allowing sufficient time for questions and discussion, and avoiding confusing messages all enhance these strategies. When English is not the family's language at home, it will be necessary to use an interpreter to ensure that all members of the family understand. Children of immigrant parents may have good use of English if they are at school, and they often interpret for their parents, but they should not be made responsible for passing on this information.

At the end of the assessment programme, the parents need time to discuss with the paediatrician the results of all the investigations. This will lead to the decision to recommend a transplant for the child, and when to be placed on the active waiting list for an organ. It may be that a transplant cannot be recommended and the reasons must be explained fully. In this situation, the family will need appropriate support from the hospital and local health professionals to enable them to give the care they wish and to ensure the child is comfortable.

Preparing the child

Careful preparation before admission is clearly vital for transplant patients, many of whom will enter hospital at short notice (Bradford and Tomlinson, 1990). The child will need to know certain basic information about what is going to happen: where she will be nursed, the wound, some details about tubes going in and out of the body and that parents will be there when she wakes after the operation. Specially adapted teddy bears, photographs and the opportunity to meet with other children who have had transplants are helpful to both patients and parents.

If children require barrier nursing after the surgery, they will need to be prepared. The hospital play specialists may make plans with the child for play around chosen themes and help to familiarise the child with gowns, masks and any special equipment. Each child and family should be considered individually as to how much detail to discuss. Some children can become upset and obsessed by details of postoperative care, such as the large wound or a drain or tube, and so would not benefit from having weeks or months during which to become increasingly anxious.

Older children have their own questions to ask and need time and privacy to discuss them. Common fears include waking up during the operation and taking on some characteristics of the donor. If the child is able to understand appropriate information and is involved in the decisions, it aids recovery and may also help the parents to cope.

Parents may need more time to consider transplantation and all the relevant issues, depending on the child's state of health. They may feel that it is not right to subject the child to such a complicated procedure and an uncertain future. On the other hand, the child may choose the way to proceed (see Case Study 10.1).

CASE STUDY 10.1   Children sometimes take the difficult decisions

Anna, aged 7, was offered a second liver transplant when her graft failed. Her mother asked what she would like to do. She replied that she wanted to go home. Her parents felt reassured that they had done as she wished, and she died peacefully at home a few days later.

THE WAITING PERIOD

The length of this period varies according to the urgency of the transplant, the length of the waiting list and the organ concerned. It should not be underestimated how stressful this time can be, particularly for the parents, but also for the child. The main stress factors at this time are listed in Box 10.1.

Box 10.1   Main stress factors whilst waiting for the transplant (Noble-Jamieson *et al.*, 1996)

- Being told that a transplant is needed
- Fear of the operation and complications
- Agonizing over the right time for the transplant
- Fear that the child may be too ill when a graft is found
- Possibility of dying before the transplant
- Bleeding from varices (in liver failure)
- Receiving different messages from different members of the team
- Perceived lack of medical expertise in the child's condition locally
- Anticipated grief and guilt for the family who will lose a child

Supporting the family during the waiting period

If the child is well enough to wait at home for the transplant, the family will still find this a very difficult period. They may feel forgotten if they are not in regular contact with the centre, and need reassurance that the child is still on the list and receiving good medical care to ensure the best chance for the operation.

There are periods of depression for some parents when they think the organ will not come in time and the child will die, and there are also times when they feel excited, happy and positive that their child will be well again soon.

Parents want their child to remain as healthy as possible (Gold *et al.*, 1986) and become anxious when the child shows any signs of deterioration. General practitioners and local health centres need to be sensitive to the parent's concerns and perhaps check with the hospital for reassurance.

It is usually helpful to remind parents about planning for the hospital admission; they should be making lists of what to bring into hospital, both for themselves and for the child; arranging to have other children and the family pets looked after, and booking time off work. When they get the telephone call informing them that a donor organ is available, there is often a moment of panic and a rush of emotion, so it is helpful to have done the planning calmly in advance.

For the single parent, the ordeal ahead may seem even more daunting. It can be lonely in hospital and the task of signing the consent form for the operation may be particularly hard without another parent to share the decision. It is often helpful for the parent to have her mother, sister or a friend to support her in hospital. In this situation, it would be helpful to offer some preparation to the companion.

Parents are often given a bleeper to take home as a way of making sure they can be contacted quickly. Some parents find this a great benefit, knowing that they can go out shopping without missing the vital telephone call. Whilst these parents will feel the bleeper gives them a freedom, others will say that they feel trapped by it. They do not like having it with them at all times, they are scared of it sounding, and above all it is a constant reminder that they are waiting for a dreadful ordeal. Parents must be warned that it may give false alarms. Some parents have said that a false alarm was reassuring, as they knew the bleeper was working and they were not forgotten. Others have told of the initial panic before ringing the hospital only to find out it was a mistake; nevertheless, it had been helpful, as they were not so shocked when it alarmed again.

Visits to hospitals a long way from home can cause considerable financial difficulties. Even if the family has a reasonably regular income, the extra costs of journeys and of living in hospital mean there is less money available to pay the usual bills. Some centres are able to give assistance from special funds and social workers can advise on the benefits to which they are entitled.

The child waiting in hospital may be very sick, possibly even in a life-threatening condition. For these families, the sense of urgency is great – Will the organ come in time to save the child; will the child be too sick to have the operation; perhaps the child will die before a transplant becomes a possibility? Parents have been heard to comment on a holiday weekend that statistically there are more accidents at weekends and holidays, so perhaps there will be some donors available. It is desperately hard for parents not to put their own child's needs first, even at the cost of others. They are then often overcome with guilt for having such thoughts. Some parents will ask about donors – where do they come from; what are the causes of death? They may need to know some facts; otherwise they may find it frustrating and confusing to be waiting for what seems like a long time when people are dying all the time.

Children may die on the waiting list; this is always sad as they did not even have the chance of a transplant. Some parents try to comfort themselves by saying that perhaps it was meant to be, and that at least the child was spared the operation, which might not have worked anyway. There may even be tremendous relief that it is all over, but also anger that the organ did not come in time.

Some families find it important to be 'doing something to help', such as inviting the media to be involved in their story, hoping that it might increase public awareness of the need for organ donors. They may join a support group or raise money for research into the child's condition, or for hospital equipment.

THE TRANSPLANT OPERATION

When parents hear that a suitable donor organ has been found for their child, the child may be at home, perhaps quite well, even at school, or she may be in hospital, possibly very sick. The family may arrive at the hospital tired after the journey and then have a short wait before the start time for the anaesthetic. An older child may like to visit the intensive care unit to be reminded of the surroundings and meet the nurses. Some like to choose the quilt covers or the music, and make special requests such as photographs to be taken whilst on the ventilator so that they can see what they looked like. This sounds strange to some adults, but it is interesting to note how many children do like photographs taken; some ask to have a piece of their old liver to keep, or a laboratory photograph of the old organ. With proper appropriate explanation, this can help the older child to understand the difference between a healthy and a diseased organ and why, therefore, the operation was necessary.

The time before going to theatre is often regarded as a special time for families and should be as calm, and perhaps private, as possible. They will be anxious, naturally, and many parents have said that they did not know whether this would be their last time with their child.

Parents usually accompany the child, with a nurse, to the theatre, but should not be made to feel guilty if this is too much for them. The responsibility of handing over the child for such major surgery is huge and they may need time to recover afterwards. Most parents have said they wanted to hold the child during anaesthetic induction, that they felt much calmer knowing they had helped their child to go to sleep with them and not with a stranger.

During the surgery, parents feel remarkably helpless – there is nothing they can do for the child. Some like to go out; it is reassuring for them if they can take the bleep so that they can be called back if needed, or they might ring the unit at regular intervals. Most parents prefer to stay nearby, trying to catch up on sleep, resting or distracting themselves by reading or watching television.

It is very helpful if, during this long wait, a member of the medical team or a transplant coordinator or specialist nurse can meet the parents at regular intervals to provide an update on how the operation is proceeding. There may not be much information available but, especially if the surgery is complicated, these meetings will ensure that parents do not feel forgotten. Some have reported that this regular contact really helped them to stay calm and helped the time to pass.

THE POSTOPERATIVE PERIOD

When the operation is over, the child is returned to the intensive care unit. After the theatre team has handed over and the unit staff have connected all the equipment and started the observations, the parents are able to come in and see their child. It is helpful if they are reminded what they will see and how the child will look before they are escorted in. First reactions vary, but staff should be prepared for a wide range of emotions. When the parents are ready, the equipment and care should be explained and time given to tell them about the operation.

The transplant operation is a turning point for the family and their lives will not be the same again. They have been awaiting this day with mixed feelings and I think that it is worth acknowledging with them how hard it has been for them. It is therefore important for them to try to rest themselves while the child is asleep on the ventilator as they will be needing renewed energies when the child starts to wake up. It may be that they need permission from the nurses to leave the unit for a break – a meal, a walk or a sleep – but knowing they can ring at any time.

The length of time in intensive care will vary according to each child, so no promises can be given. The parents often feel euphoric after the child has survived the surgery and get excited about planning ahead, but they need to remain cautious – there are many complications and problems that can occur. In fact, it is often when the first problem happens that the parents' 'brave face' falls apart as the repressed emotion is released.

Information about the child's progress is important for most families and some become quite obsessed by test results. Some parents do not find it helpful to be given detailed information and prefer simply to be told if the child is better or worse. Uncertainty is always difficult and parents should be encouraged to take, not one day, but a few hours at a time. It is helpful if warning can be given in advance of planned or possible tests or procedures.

When the child is well enough to be transferred to the high-dependency area and then to the ward, the parents are able to carry out more of the child's care themselves. Being away from intensive care nursing may be a relief to parents, knowing that the child must be getting better, but they can also feel the loss of constant attention from nursing and medical staff.

Complications, particularly infection and rejection, may occur and other problems such as difficulties with feeding may cause parents' moods to swing continually. Changes in the child's condition during relatively short periods produce this 'roller coaster' effect (Gold *et al.*, 1986).

The aim throughout this period and afterwards must be for the child to be treated as normally as possible. This means a normal diet leading to normal growth and development for the age, normal activities and a normal structure to each day. Many parents find it very difficult to establish boundaries and discipline after the child has had a transplant, but this is an important element in the rehabilitation and they need support and encouragement. If the child is of school age, it should be possible to start some school work from the hospital teacher or the child's school, otherwise the return to school may be more traumatic if much time has been missed.

Discharge home

Most parents are secretly longing to be allowed to go home, but at the same time are likely to be daunted by the thought of caring for the child on their own again. Planning for discharge needs to be considered carefully. If a date is given too far ahead, a problem may occur which could delay the discharge and cause the family to become upset. On the other hand, they will need time to prepare both practically and psychologically.

It is often helpful for the family to stay off the ward for a few days or to go home for a weekend if they live near enough. This gives them time to build their confidence with giving new medication and a new diet, knowing they are in touch with the hospital. Parents often describe a feeling of taking a new baby home again, which in some ways it is. One mother even commented that she hoped she would like the 'new' child she had exchanged, and that they would need a period to get to know each other.

For some families, this period of adapting to the new situation is far from easy. It may take some time for siblings to accept the child back into the family. The child who was sick and needed so much of the parents' time and attention is back at home and may not be too welcome at first. One little girl was so used to her twin being weaker that she was really shocked when she was hit by her – this twin was different from the one she remembered!

It is not uncommon for parents of children who have received transplants to suffer a period of depression some time after discharge home. This is perhaps a necessary part of the adaptation to the new situation, a sort of resting time when they are not able to cope with anything more in their lives until they have settled this one big issue. A great deal has happened to them and their family and they are probably emotionally exhausted. Some parents find it helpful to talk through their memories of the child's illness, diagnosis, time in hospital, problems at home, time in intensive care and thoughts of the donor before they can move on to thinking about their worries for the future (see Case Study 10.2).

CASE STUDY 10.2   Adapting to the discharge home

The mother of a child who had a liver transplant after an acute illness found herself unable to bear comments from relations and friends such as 'You must be over the moon that she is well again' and 'It's a miracle how well she is, everything will be fine now'. Of course, the mother was extremely grateful to the hospitals for making her child better, but part of her was also saying: 'But I did not want my child to be critically ill, let alone have a transplant. I just wanted everything to be back how it was before.' For this very capable and caring mother the grief at the loss of her normal child needed to be acknowledged, and the controlled anger she admitted was part of her grieving. She needed time to talk about these feelings, which she and her husband had found difficult to manage. Her husband also found it helpful to talk about how he was feeling; it helped him to know that his wife was having support from the team who understood them.

LONG-TERM MANAGEMENT

The future is uncertain for all children who have received transplants. Some organs have a longer-term success than others and they all have their own specific problems and complications. The quality of the child's life has to be the most important factor, but the way in which the family adapts is also critical. There are now many children who are enjoying full and happy lives after transplantation, taking part in active sports, achieving well at school, some even reaching university. However, most parents will always have some fears for the future, no matter how well their child appears to be.

A study of children by Zitelli *et al.* (1988) noted that, overall, objective changes in lifestyle as well as parents' perceptions of behaviour of children appear to be improved after liver transplantation.

Regular hospital visits

The importance of following the advice of the hospital team cannot be underestimated and good communication with the child's local hospital and general practitioner are part of this. Blood tests to check the levels of immunosuppression are vital; other checks may include ultrasound scans and tests for the normal functioning of the transplanted organ.

Parents often enjoy returning to the transplant centre and find the reassurance a necessary element in their coping. It is rewarding for the team to see children who are well some years after transplantation and gives them encouragement in this sensitive and sometimes controversial field of treatment.

Psychosocial aspects after transplantation

Consultations need to focus not only on medical aspects, but also on more general issues, such as how the family are coping and whether the child's development is appropriate for age, as it is only in integrating psychosocial and medical factors that optimal care can be provided (Bradford and Tomlinson, 1990).

Given the degree of stress these children have faced and the fact that the diagnosis of a possible terminal illness is likely to have a significant negative impact on psychological functioning, it would be surprising to find no residual effects (Windsorova *et al.*, 1991). A paediatric team that is aware of psychosocial issues will be able to meet many of the needs of transplant patients, but should be able to make specific referrals where appropriate (Reynolds *et al.*, 1991).

Education and social development

The child's growth, social and intellectual development should be assessed regularly and matters such as school progress need to be discussed. Many of these children have missed large periods of school time or have not caught up with the development of their peers by the time they should start school. Extra help from teachers, school helpers and parents may be needed, and some children benefit from being in a class a year below their age.

There may have to be some restrictions on the child's physical activities, which unfortunately sets the child aside from peers, but there are other opportunities to encourage the child to join in recreation and make friends.

Overprotection

After the ordeal of a transplant, it is not easy for parents to try to treat the child 'normally' – parents talk about 'wrapping him in cotton wool' and not wanting to let him out of their sight. Schools find it hard to know what to expect from the child and need to have clear guidelines from the medical team in agreement with parents.

It is a huge step for parents to allow the child to go away on the first school day out or on holiday. It helps to give written information about the child's medication, any dietary restrictions and contact telephone numbers in case of illness or questions. The parent's natural anxiety needs to be recognised; sometimes they can laugh about it, but they may be quite frightened at letting go of the child's care. When the child returns and all is well, the parents feel a relief and reassurance.

Starting school is another big hurdle, particularly for mothers, and many parents telephone the hospital just to check that it is all right. The fear of the child picking up infections at school is a constant worry at first, and some immunosuppressed children need medication if they are in contact with chickenpox.

Advice for families going on holiday, particularly abroad, is important. Children taking immunosuppressive drugs cannot have live vaccines. It is advisable to take a letter from the hospital giving details of the child's treatment, particularly the current medications, and a contact telephone number for advice in an emergency. Sufficient supplies of medication should be taken, and sometimes a letter explaining why the child needs the drugs is helpful to prevent problems with customs.

CONSIDERATIONS AS THE CHILD GROWS UP

As children grow older, they will hopefully develop responsibility for themselves. Children who have had transplants have additional problems as well as the usual ones of their peers, such as the change in body image – possibly the side-effects of immunosuppressive drugs and steroids such as increased body hair, swollen gums or change in face shape. The large scar may be an embarrassment for girls, but I know one boy who is a keen swimmer and tells his friends that the scar resulted from a shark attack!

Future problems may include difficulties with higher education and vocational training if school achievement has been poor, although many children have reached high academic levels. Employers are not always sympathetic to time off for regular hospital visits, and life assurance may not be possible.

COMPLIANCE

Adolescents sometimes do have problems complying with treatment for any condition, so it is not just transplanted children who may rebel. Unfortunately, it can cause irreversible damage if immunosuppression is stopped. Regular blood tests to show that therapeutic levels of the drugs are being maintained should identify any cause for concern. It is vital that teenagers understand the importance of regular medication and blood tests. They may be helped by making charts to record their medication and by having their own written information as well as their parents.

DEATH OF A CHILD

Although the numbers of children who survive a transplant have increased significantly over recent years, children die on the waiting list for organs, and others may die soon after or from complications some time after the transplant operation. Having gone through such a major operation, it is extremely sad to lose the child, both for the family and for the professionals who have worked hard for the child and on whom the family have placed so much hope. Other parents feel the loss too; many families become close through meeting in hospital or one of the support organisations. They know only too well that their child could die and another child's death may affect them deeply.

CONCLUSION

Controversies and discussions continue around the subject of organ donation and transplantation, often creating difficulties and confusion for families. Professionals working in this field need to be well informed and very sensitive to the feelings and fears of the children and their families.

Transplantation is still a relatively new treatment and, although the long-term survival rate is higher for some organs than for others, the future is not certain. The surgical skills and postoperative management improve with experience, and although the survival time may lengthen in years, new problems will arise to challenge the knowledge and experience of the professionals. It is not surprising that parents continue to be anxious about their child's future.

There are an increasing number of families who are grateful for their child's transplant and the quality of life they are now able to enjoy. We must not, however, underestimate the high level of support they need from health professionals and others, throughout all the stages of their long ordeal.

REFERENCES

Alderson, P. (1993) *Children's Consent to Surgery.* Buckingham: Open University Press.

Beauchamp, T. L. & Childress, J. F. (1994) *Principles of Biomedical Ethics,* 4th edn. New York: Oxford University Press.

Bradford, R. & Tomlinson, L. (1990) Psychological guidelines in the management of paediatric organ transplantation. *Archives of Disease in Childhood,* **65,** 1000–1003.

Castledine, G. (1993) Laura Davies: should children always get the treatment they need? *British Journal of Nursing,* **2(21),** 1077–1078.

Children Act, The (1989: England and Wales; 1995: Scotland). London: HMSO

Cook, P. (1996) Long term follow-up and support. In *Working with Children in Grief and Loss,* ed. Lindsay, B. & Elsegood, J, Ch. 6. London: Baillière Tindall.

Froment, P. (1992) Hope and fear: the paradox. **Nursing, 5(2),** 13–14.

Gillon, R. (1996) Transplantation and ethics. In: *Birth to Death,* ed. Thomasma, D. C. & Kushner, T. Cambridge: Cambridge University Press.

Gold, L. M., Kirkpatrick, B. S., Fricker, F. J. & Zitelli, B. J. (1986) Psychosocial issues in pediatric organ transplantation: the parents' perspective. *Pediatrics,* **77,** 738–743.

Maynard, L. (1993) Transplantation in children: psychological issues. *Paediatric Nursing,* **5(10),** 20–22.

Noble-Jamieson, G., Cook, P., Parkinson, G. & Barnes, N. (1996) Coping strategies in parents of children receiving liver transplants. *Clinical Child Psychology and Psychiatry,* **1,** 563–573.

Reynolds, J. M., Garralda, M. E., Postlethwaite, R. J. & Goh, D. (1991) Changes in psychological adjustment after renal transplantation. *Archives of Disease in Childhood,* **66,** 508–513.

Warner, J. O. (1991) Heart-lung transplantation: all the facts. *Archives of Disease in Childhood,* **66,** 1013–1017.

Windsorova, D., Stewart, S. M., Lovitt, R., Waller, D. A. & Andrews, W. S. (1991) Emotional adaptation in children after liver transplantation. *Journal of Pediatrics,* **119,** 880–887.

Zitelli, B. J., Miller, J. W., Gartner, J. C., Malatack, J. J., Urbach, A. H., Belle, S. H., Williams, L., Kirkpatrick, B. & Starzl, T. E. (1988) Changes in lifestyle after liver transplantation. *Pediatrics,* **82,** 173–180.

Siblings of sick children

INTRODUCTION

Brothers and sisters have special relationships within families, which may not be recognised by the parents. Sometimes they appear to show great love for each other, but at others intense hate. There may be jealousy, resentment and rivalry or competition for parents' attentions. Even though the children may be brought up by the same parents, usually in the same home, with similar family values and outlook on life, children will develop their own individual thoughts and view of the world, because it is different for each one. There are many factors to do with being a sibling which influence the life of a sibling, such as:

- sex of child – e.g. the only boy among girls, one of many girls
- age – may be too young to play with an older sibling, of a similar age or much older
- place in family – may be, for example, youngest, eldest, half-brother, step-sister
- common interests with another sibling – e.g. they play football together, attend the same school
- being a twin or one of triplets – twins and triplets have special relationships often unknown to adults.

If a child has a brother or sister who is ill or injured, this is yet another factor which will have an influence. The siblings of a chronically or terminally ill child are often forced to take a back seat when the sibling needs constant attention (Cook, 1996). Changes have to be made to the normal family routines, the parents are unlikely to be their usual selves, as they are anxious, and the priorities will have changed. It has been found that in chronic and lifethreatening conditions, there is a significant response by siblings of the sick child (Hewitt, 1990). The two main areas identified are practical consequences of the disability or illness, and relationships within the family; these are discussed in the section on siblings' needs (p. 141).

SIBLINGS' REACTIONS TO A CHILD'S ILLNESS

Relationships within families and communication patterns are important factors in determining how siblings react to a brother's or sister's illness; the type and severity of illness are not such reliable indicators (Muller, Harris & Wattley, 1986). It is easier for children to adapt to having a sick sibling in a family in which it is usual to discuss matters openly and to share feelings and emotions. How well the parents are coping will also have an effect on how the children are managing the changes in the family circumstances.

Rosen (1986) wrote that it is clear that brothers and sisters of children with cancer and other life-threatening conditions experience a variety of problems resulting from the tragic circumstances of their lives, noting that failure to thrive, irritability and withdrawal are among the more common of these.

Reasons for stress and changes in behaviour of siblings of hospitalised children are thought to be related to parental preoccupation with the ill child, the stress the parents are experiencing and the separation that occurs between parents and siblings when the ill child is admitted to hospital (Morrison, 1997). Other stresses for the children should also be considered as they may have a significant effect on their way of coping. These might include:

- parent's separation
- changing school
- moving house
- death of a pet
- bullying
- pressure of schoolwork.

Physical symptoms of a child's distress may develop, such as feeling generally tired and unwell, nausea, vomiting, diarrhoea, constipation, headache and aching limbs. Symptoms connected with the sick sibling's condition may also be reported. The child needs to be understood and not made to feel that the fears have been dismissed as unimportant (see Case Study 11.1).

CASE STUDY 11.1   *Physical reaction to a sibling's illness*

Daniel was 10 years old when his older brother suffered a brain haemorrhage; he became very frightened and complained of headaches. Fortunately his mother discussed this with the hospital team and the doctor paid special attention to reassuring Daniel.

Behavioural changes may include unusual aggression, temper or withdrawal from family or friends, rudeness, bullying and demanding attention. Regression in the form of thumb-sucking, bed-wetting, clinging, eating problems or school refusal may be noticed. Sleeping problems could include a fear of the dark, nightmares, waking in the night and wanting to sleep in the parents' bed.

SIBLINGS' NEEDS

Two of the most important needs for siblings of a sick child are *to be informed* and *to be involved*. This means they need to be told, in language appropriate for their age and in a simple but honest way, some facts about the illness, such as:

- What is the matter with the child – what is the illness called?
- Where is the child – which hospital?
- Who is looking after the child?
- What is being done to make the illness/injury better?
- When can they visit?
- When will the child be coming home?
- Why did it happen?
- Will it happen to me too?
- How does this affect me?

Parents and other relatives and friends may try to shelter the siblings from the truth, particularly if the illness is serious or unpleasant, or the injuries severe. This protection from the truth only increases fears and fantasies, which may be far worse than what is really happening to their brother or sister.

The importance of including siblings in the care of children awaiting surgery should not be ignored. Warning parents of possible behaviour problems, helping them to provide coping strategies, increasing siblings' involvement in the care and reducing their misunderstandings are part of the responsibilities of health professionals.

The most important source of support should ideally be from the parents, but this may not be easy if a child is admitted to hospital in an emergency or if they need to be with the sick child. Parents, or whoever is taking on the role of caring for the siblings, have a responsibility to keep them informed and involved, which means giving them support by telling them what is happening to the sick child and to them, answering their questions and admitting when they do not know the answers. By not keeping the truth from siblings, their fears will be reduced and hopefully they will be encouraged to share their feelings with the adults.

Siblings need their own emotional support

Children need adults to talk to them, but also to listen to them. Siblings may be sensitive to their parents' emotions and try to protect them from any more hurt or worries, and so may bottle up their own feelings instead of sharing them. Parents may be so 'busy' with the sick child that they feel unable to take on the emotional support of their other children.

Feelings that need to be understood include:

- resentment – that the sick child is taking so much of the parents' time and attention
- jealousy – the sick child is given presents and does not have to do schoolwork
- isolation – through being separated from parents, cared for by others and not being told what is happening
- fear – of what they do not know; of death (of sibling or themselves)
- guilt – that it could perhaps be their fault in some way; for having bad feelings
- anger – that this is happening in their family; towards the sibling for being sick
- despair – that life will never get better.

Siblings need to see their parents

It is helpful if parents are able to spend time at home with the children, particularly at times of the day when they would normally be there. Perhaps someone else will be able to visit the sick child sometimes, so that a parent can meet the other children from school and hear about their day's activities, or be there for teatime or bedtime. Parents usually feel a need to see their well children, so time with them is beneficial for all. Some parents are fortunate to have good support from family and friends to enable them to plan time with each child.

Keeping the normal family routine

Familiar routines are important for children's sense of security and it is reassuring if they can be maintained as far as possible. This includes going to school, giving a normal structure to the day and maintaining their education and contact with their own peer group.

Siblings need to feel in touch with the sick child when they cannot visit

A photograph of the sick child for siblings to keep is often appreciated. It could be a family photograph, when the child was well, or an instant picture taken in hospital. Photographs of babies in a neonatal unit remind the family that they do have a baby; brothers and sisters can look at it and see that their baby has to grow bigger and stronger before being able to come home (see Case Study 11.2).

CASE STUDY 11.2   Photographs help siblings to feel in touch

Shaun was 5 when his brother was taken to hospital after being knocked over by a car. His mother explained that he was in a special part of the hospital called intensive care where the doctors and nurses were going to make him better. Shaun said he would help Mummy look after him, and wondered why he couldn't come home. His mother showed him the instant photograph taken by the nurse and pointed out the equipment around his bed. Shaun's immediate comment was: 'Of course he can't come home yet – we couldn't fit all that lot in our bedroom!'

Some siblings really need to know where the sick child is living

Siblings may already know the hospital and may be able to visualise the ward, but if they do not, they may have fantasies about it (see Case Study 11.3).

CASE STUDY 11.3   Siblings may need to see the sick child's room

Emma was 9 when her younger brother was in intensive care for 2 days after an operation. She wanted to come to the hospital with her parents, but when they arrived at the ward she could not face going in to see him with tubes attached. She chose to stay in the playroom on the ward and drew him a picture with his name on to put up over his bed. The nurse looking after her brother went to see her in the playroom and introduced herself as his nurse and explained why he needed to be in the unit. She showed her the door to his room so that she knew exactly where he was and who was with him.

Siblings can visit the sick child in hospital

The child patient looks forward to seeing people from outside the world of the hospital, particularly family members, including the siblings where possible. When we watch children with their brothers and sisters, we can usually see that they have a special relationship that no one else can match. Parents often comment that siblings argue or fight at home but are reassured that, when one of them is ill, the others show their concern.

Siblings are good at telling sick children in hospital about their pets and special toys; they need to know they are being cared for while they are not at home. They are also often able to play normally together within the restrictions of hospital treatment, which is sometimes helpful in the sick child's rehabilitation (see case study 11.4).

CASE STUDY 11.4   *Through play, siblings can encourage 'normality'*

Simon had a damaged hand and the physiotherapist wanted him to use it as much as he could even though it was bandaged. He was very reluctant to lift it out from under the bedclothes because he did not like looking at it. It was interesting to notice how he started to move his hand while his sister was visiting him. She brought him some of his favourite toy cars, and they began to play with them on the bed table. His sister had been told about his hand and was not surprised or upset when she saw it. It is possible that Simon had been reassured when his sister accepted his hand without comment and that this helped him to become more confident. He was certainly very pleased to play with his cars, and his sister had enabled him to be quite natural with her and to play normally.

Sometimes the siblings need to know that they have a choice about visiting the hospital; it might be too distressing or they might simply prefer to go to a friend's house to play.

Siblings imagine that the same thing may happen to them

It is not unreasonable for young children who live in the same household and who are treated equally by the parents to believe that they will suffer the same problems as their sick sibling. They need to be reassured that this is not the case, and given an explanation as to why it will not happen to them too.

CASE STUDY 11.5   *Will it happen to me too?*

James was 5 when his older brother of 7 was being treated for leukaemia. During one of the hospital visits, he asked the doctor if he would also get leukaemia when he was 7.

Siblings need to know when the sick child is coming home again

The knowledge that a sick child will be coming home at some time in the future is an important indicator to siblings that life may return to normal – at least all the family members will be living together once again. They may stay somewhere else when a parent is at the hospital with the sick child. It is wiser not to be definite about dates unless they are certain; children may not understand a change of plan or in the condition of the child. It is more likely to confuse them and decrease their trust in the adults around them.

Siblings often ask: why did this happen?

There are often unspoken fears among siblings that what has happened to their brother or sister will happen to them too. Sometimes they may even believe that they have caused it in some way. Adults need to be careful to reassure children that there was nothing they did that could have caused this illness or accident. This question can also be considered alongside others: what is wrong; what is the illness called? Simple explanations to answer a child's questioning must be honest and must be under-stood by the child. This information will be built on as the sibling finds out more and as the circumstances change. This is especially important if the sick child's condition deteriorates, or if he becomes terminally ill and dies.

SUPPORT GROUPS FOR SIBLINGS OF SICK CHILDREN

Some wards or units for children arrange special days or groups for siblings of sick children in their care. These are especially helpful for families of children with serious life-threatening or life-limiting conditions, such as cancer, liver disease, or physical or learning difficulties. One hospital (Stone, 1993) decided to set up a group for siblings of children with cancer, with the following aims:

- to make siblings feel special
- to educate them on the disease, tests and treatment
- to enable them to discuss their feelings on their brother's or sister's diagnosis of cancer and its effect on them and their family.

Not all children benefit from groups and some will decide definitely not to attend. Other important issues to consider include venue, days and times, which children to invite, activi-ties, refreshments, funding and sufficient helpers. The staff should probably include nurses with a good knowledge of the condition(s) and experience of treatments, and play specialists.

SUPPORT FROM SCHOOL

It is helpful for the siblings of sick children if their school teachers are kept informed about the sick child's condition. The teachers may observe changes in behaviour or attention. They may also be asked questions about the illness by siblings, and so usually like to be prepared for this. A class teacher who is well known to the child could become a trusted source of support outside the family. The school nurse may also be able to help with the child's understanding of the illness and talk about fears and thoughts.

THE DEATH OF A SIBLING

The death of a sibling has a profound effect on children, sometimes taking many months or years to resolve. Because children look to their parents to keep them safe, the loss of a family member heightens their sense of vulnerability (Jewett, 1982). Some future problems can be avoided if the children are encouraged to be involved with their dying sibling, such as:

- helping with care, visiting in hospital, playing, reading a story
- asking questions to understand what is happening and to be reassured about pain
- sharing feelings with adults, seeing adults cry.

McGowan (1994) found that one of the most significant perspectives to be identified in the literature was the importance of measuring the sibling's personal experience and not relying on parental insight, which is often incorrect. He also found that involving the siblings in the child's care enables them to have the opportunity for anticipatory mourning and gradual preparation, thus making the death less frightening.

A study by Pettle Michael and Lansdown (1986) highlighted the importance of children's perceptions of themselves and their world, and of recognising that they cannot be seen as merely being on the receiving end of events or guided by their parents' inability to cope with trauma. They concluded that excluding children from information is unsuccessful in reducing their pain, as clearly they sense that something is seriously amiss and, in the absence of age-appropriate explanations, are prone to fantasise.

Children are much more able to deal with difficult situations when they know the facts; otherwise they will make them up, and their fantasies may be worse than the truth. One teenager, for example, asked to see her brother after he had died because she wanted 'to see what they had done to him'. She was relieved to see that he looked peaceful and that nothing dreadful had 'been done' to him. It is well worth taking the time to talk with the children, as it makes them feel included in what is happening, but they must be well supported throughout (see Case study 11.6).

CASE STUDY 11.6   Giving siblings the facts

Michael was a mature 10-year-old asking sensible questions about his sister's head injuries. The neurosurgeon showed him the scans of his sister's head, which showed the large areas of bleeding and brain swelling. He explained what was wrong and why she could not recover. Michael was naturally upset, but he understood why his sister was going to die and could share with his parents the feelings they had.

If siblings are not present at the death, they need to be told what has happened soon afterwards, by someone whom they know and trust. They need to be told the truth, in words they can understand, building on what they already know. They will want to know that everything was done to try to make their sibling better, that it did not hurt and that it is not going to happen to them as well. They will need the reassurance that the other people in their lives are still there for them, and still want to care for them.

Older children may like to be involved in a decision about organ donation. They may have discussed the subject at school and may even carry their own donor card. There is something rather special about a sibling sharing in giving permission for organ donation. In addition, it may be comforting for parents to know that their decision had been approved.

Children who are old enough to understand will need to be able to believe what they are being told, so it is usually important for them to have the chance to say goodbye. They will then see for themselves that the sibling looks different, but at the same time it can be explained that all is peaceful. A child should not be forced to kiss a brother or sister; there are other ways of saying goodbye such as writing a note, leaving a toy with the body or having a few moments alone to say something special (see Case Study 11.7).

CASE STUDY 11.7   Allowing siblings the opportunity to say goodbye

Sanjo was 12 when his sister died after a long-term disability. When he came to the hospital to see her in the chapel of rest, he brought a flower to lay beside her. It was explained to him that she looked pale and would be cold, but that he could touch her if he wanted to. He chose to go with the nurse and asked his mother to wait in the adjoining room. When he was with his sister, he asked the nurse if people in the next room could hear what was being said in the chapel. The nurse asked if that was important to him, and when he replied that it was, she asked him if that meant he would like to be alone with his sister for a moment. She promised she would wait just outside the door and return for him in 2 minutes unless he came out first. It was clear that Sanjo had something important to say to his sister that he did not want his mother to hear. Later on, his mother said that sometimes Sanjo was not very kind to his sister; her disability had affected his life too. Perhaps he needed to say he was sorry to her.

Survivor guilt

There is often a feeling of guilt among those who have lost a person close to them through death. This is particularly so within families, especially among grandparents, who think it should be members of their generation who die, not their grandchildren. Siblings sometimes feel strongly that they should have been the one to die; this may have to do with a feeling that the dead child was the favourite, or was more attractive or more clever, and that the parents will miss him more. The accompanying sense of guilt, the 'survivor guilt' can be quite overwhelming. In cases where a sibling has been involved in the death, this sense of guilt may be compounded by feelings of responsibility (see Case Study 11.8).

CASE STUDY 11.8   Survivor guilt and feelings of responsibility

A brother and sister had an argument before they got off the school bus. They did not cross the road together, and the brother rushed out from behind the bus and was hit by a lorry. He died in intensive care the next day. His sister felt very responsible for the accident and it took a considerable amount of careful talking with her before she was able to see him in hospital. Some later counselling sessions enabled her to talk about what had happened. She had witnessed the death of her brother and had to adapt to life without him.

Sometimes the situation might allow other people to blame a sibling for what happened; indeed, it may well have been the sibling's fault, indirectly if not directly. The bereaved child will have to live with the memory of this terrible event and its consequences, so it is helpful to be able to find parts of the story which allow the child to be 'let off' some of the responsibility (see Case Study 11.9).

> **CASE STUDY 11.9**   *Finding something positive to help the survivor*
>
> Matthew and his brother Chris were both on Matthew's bicycle going downhill at considerable speed when the front wheel hit a large stone. Both boys fell off the bicycle but Chris was catapulted and landed on his head. Neither of the boys was wearing a protective helmet; Chris sustained severe head injuries and was rushed to hospital and the intensive care unit. He died a few days later with all his family around him.
>
> Matthew sat beside Chris in hospital for most of the day and frequently mumbled that he should have been the one lying there: it was his fault, he had been in control of the bicycle and had killed his brother. There were other factors to consider as well as not wearing helmets, which their parents had told them to wear always. The boys were supposed to be doing school work and had not told anyone they were going out. They had known that two of them should not be on one bicycle, and they had been riding where it was not permitted.
>
> Amid the powerful feelings of guilt that Matthew felt, blaming himself for the accident, he also felt there was disapproval coming from other people, who must be blaming him too. He became more morose and withdrawn, saying that he wanted to die and be with Chris. This was a tragic accident which would not have happened 'if only' the boys had been doing their school work, if they had not been cycling where they were not allowed, and if they were not going fast with two on the bicycle; furthermore, head injuries would not have been so severe if only they had worn helmets.
>
> All of these facts had to be acknowledged, but there were a few points to help Matthew in some small way. When he told his story of the events leading to the accident, it was revealed that Chris had asked Matthew to take out his bike and begged him to let him ride on the back. Chris had persuaded Matthew to go fast and had been shouting in delight and excitement just before the crash. After some time talking about this in private, Matthew was able to feel that perhaps this tragedy was not solely his fault and that Chris had been partly responsible. This helped him to feel relieved of some of the heavy responsibility. He recognised that as Chris had been unconscious from the moment his head hit the road, his last moments were happy and carefree, having fun with Matthew, who now believed he died happy.

HOME

Life at home can never be the same again after the death of a child. When a sibling is missing, the normal roles within a family change, adding to the confusion and uncertainty. Parents are often so deep in their own grief that they are unable to give the remaining children the attention they need. Hutton and Bradley (1994) commented that few studies of parental reactions to sudden infant death have included a comparison group. Therefore, most studies cannot tell us to what extent the symptoms of illness and disruptions to family life are significantly different from those in families with still-living babies. The parents need to struggle with their own grief, which takes time. They are not the way they were, towards each other or towards the children (Cook, 1996). Children may try to protect the parents from any further hurt by not revealing how they are feeling or by refraining from asking the questions for which they need answers.

The change in behaviour of bereaved siblings is often hard for the parents to manage, and this can become a focus for the parents' anger and resentment away from the death of the child. Jewett (1982) considered the remaining children's changed behaviour to be a result of the changed behaviour of the parents towards them rather than a result of the death itself.

It is easy to see how parents can idolise the dead child, but what does this do for the surviving siblings? There may be many photographs of the child who died displayed around the home, but how many are there of the other children? Some parents have difficulty in changing the child's bedroom; it holds strong memories for them, containing the child's possessions and even smells of the child. When parents want to keep the room intact, perhaps with the clothes and toys still there, there is a danger that it will become a shrine. This sends very strange messages to brothers and sisters – why do we keep this room like this? The child is not here anymore, but perhaps he is coming back? It can be helpful for parents if another child asks to move into the dead child's room, as it gives them permission to change the room without letting down the child who died.

It may help younger children to understand that the sibling is not coming back if they are asked to choose, or are given, a toy or something that belonged to the child, which they can keep. A parent could ask: 'I wondered if you would like to have John's teddy bear now as he will not need it anymore.' Children will enjoy making a memory book in which they can put photographs, write stories about family events and memories of their brother or sister. A memory box is another idea for keeping small objects and pictures.

SCHOOL

Support and understanding from the siblings' school may be essential to aid their natural grieving. School may be a safer place than elsewhere for the children to talk about their feelings and what happened. A teacher, who is known and liked by the child, or the school nurse, might be able to help the children. School life is special to the child as parents usually only visit briefly, so children may like to discuss and participate in the decision as to how far within the school the information should go (Elliot,

1997). It may be possible for teachers to make links with other children who have suffered bereavement in the family and enable them to share in a group.

Nursery school teachers and play group leaders may also have in their care a young child bereaved of a sibling. Among this age group, it might be the loss of a baby through miscarriage, stillbirth, prematurity or neonatal death due, for example, to a congenital problem. The child who was looking forward to helping with a baby brother or sister is confused and unsettled. Wiltsher (1997) suggested that childcare professionals need to work closely with a child's family to help the child through the grieving process:

> The key point is to be sensitive and aware of the bereavement, to watch the child and support him through his grief, even though he may not be expressing it in an obvious way.

SUPPORT GROUPS FOR BEREAVED SIBLINGS

Groups for bereaved children are offered in some areas; they may be set up in schools, through hospitals or through a voluntary organisation such as CRUSE Bereavement Care. Experience of bereaved siblings groups organised by a hospital has shown that this can be very helpful to the children and, in turn, to their parents. If the parents attend a group for bereaved parents, they will often be keen for the children to join a group.

One of the advantages of inviting bereaved siblings to a group organised by the hospital is that there is already a link – the very important fact that the hospital staff know what happened and may be familiar to them. If the child died at home, the siblings may have had some connection with the hospital. A children's hospice has reported positive feedback from pilot schemes of groups for bereaved siblings (Gillance *et al.*, 1997). Although involvement with the whole family is essential, it showed that when children are offered time and space, shown respect, valued as individuals and given honest answers to difficult questions, these have the potential to support them in their own personal grief and life ahead.

The group must be planned carefully. Not all children benefit from a group and some will decide definitely not to attend. Some parents are wary of people outside the family being involved in their family's grief. Issues to consider include:

• *Venue* – a room suitable in size for the expected number of children and planned activities, with toilet facilities, catering arrangements, outside play and parking for parents.

- *Dates* – day; in school holidays or on Saturdays; times to start and finish; numbers of meetings.
- *Staff and helpers* – sufficient for the number of children, considering their ages and the planned activities. These will most likely include nurses, social workers, counsellors, play specialists with good understanding of children's grief and age-related reactions. It is important for all the helpers to know in advance the causes of the siblings' deaths and any relevant information, such as whether the child witnessed the death or was not involved at all.
- *Which children to invite.* Consider the ages and length of time since the death. Decide whether parents are to be included in any part of the day.
- *Activities* – Should be suitable for ages of group members and carried out in smaller groups. Equipment will be needed for games and activities such as drawing, painting, modelling and making memory books.
- *Food and drinks.*
- *Insurance.*

The children are given the opportunity to spend time with other bereaved children and to talk about their brother or sister. They have fun with games and a picnic lunch as well as therapeutic activities. These include making things for keeping special memories, offering a chance to say what they meant to say, asking questions, encouraging bad feelings such as anger to be expressed safely. It is interesting to observe how much anger some of these children are experiencing when they draw targets for their anger and then throw clay bombs at them. Common targets at which anger is directed include:

- the doctors or the hospital for not making their sibling better
- parents or grandparents for not paying as much attention to them or for not understanding them
- the school or particular teachers for not understanding them, and for telling them they should be 'over it' by now
- the treatment that the child had to endure, such as medicines, injections, drips
- other children at school who tease them about the death or say horrid things
- something or someone they can blame for the death, such as a speeding car driver or the bicycle brakes which failed
- the child who died, for causing all this upset.

When talking with these children, strong feelings of anger may emerge which need to be acknowledged, and ways of dealing with them can be discussed. Many children are angry that this terrible event happened to their sibling and to their family: 'Other children get knocked over but get better, so why did my brother have to die?' An older sibling may try to do something to address the situation such as collecting signatures on a petition to introduce speed limits or road safety posters about cycle helmets. Most children are helped by opportunities for strenuous activities – running, football, cycling – which burn up some of the energy otherwise available for angry and aggressive responses. Creative activities such as painting, modelling, playing musical instruments and making scrapbooks also help to channel the anger safely.

CONCLUSION

Health professionals working with sick children and their parents must also consider their brothers and sisters whenever possible. These children need understanding and support during a period of their lives when they may be confused, frightened, isolated and ignored.

The brothers and sisters of a sick child or a child who dies may never be able to return to normal life as they knew it before. They will have been deeply affected in many ways; children who are old enough at the time of the death to be aware of the events and emotions will remember the experiences. The child who is bereaved of a sibling will grow up to be an adult more aware of the fragility of life than most people, but with good enough support from those around, he or she will survive. Adults close to these vulnerable young people must take seriously the responsibility for their good survival.

REFERENCES

Cook, P. (1996) Long term follow-up and support. In *Working with Children in Grief and Loss*, ed. Lindsay, B. & Elsegood, J. Ch. 6. London: Baillière Tindall.

Elliot, P. (1997) *Coping with Loss for Parents. How to Help Your Child Series*. London: Piccadilly Press.

Gillance, H., Tucker, A., Aldridge, J. & Wright, J. B. (1997) Bereavement: providing support for siblings. *Paediatric Nursing*, 9(5), 22–24.

Hewitt, J. (1990) The sibling response to hospitalisation. *Paediatric Nursing*, 3, 12.

Hutton, C. J. & Bradley, B. S. (1994) Effects of sudden infant death on bereaved siblings: a comparative study. *Journal of Child Psychology and Psychiatry*, 35(4), 723–732.

Jewett, C. (1982) *Helping Children Cope with Separation and Loss*. London: Batsford.

McGowan, H. (1994) Siblings and death: perspectives and perceptions. *Paediatric Nursing,* **6(5),** 10–13.

Morrison, L. (1997) Stress and siblings. *Paediatric Nursing,* **9(4),** 26–27.

Muller, D., Harris, P. & Wattley, L. (1986) *Nursing Children: Psychology, Research and Practice.* London: Harper and Row.

Pettle Michael, S. A. & Lansdown, R. G. (1986) Adjustment to the death of a sibling. *Archives of Disease in Childhood,* **61,** 278–283.

Rosen, H. (1986) *Unspoken Grief – Coping with Childhood Sibling Loss.* Lexington: Lexington Books.

Stone, M. (1993) Lending an ear to the unheard – the role of support groups for siblings of children with cancer. *Child Health,* **1,** 54–58.

Wiltsher, A. (1997) Wiping the tears. *Nursery World,* May, 16–17.

FURTHER READING

Atkinson, N. & Crawforth, M. (1995) *All in the Family: Siblings and Disability.* London: NCH–Action for children.

Dominic, K. (1993) Left out in the cold: anxieties faced by siblings of paediatric oncology patients. *Paediatric Nursing,* **5(3),** 28–29.

Hill, L. (ed.) (1994) *Caring for Dying Children and their Families.* London: Chapman and Hall.

Lansdown, R. (1996) *Children in Hospital – a Guide for Family and Carers.* Oxford: Oxford University Press.

Lindsay, B. & Elsegood, J. (eds) (1996) *Working with Children in Grief and Loss.* London: Baillière Tindall.

Mikkelsen, J. (1993) Sibling care. In *Advances in Child Health Nursing,* ed. Glasper, E. A. & Tucker, A. London: Scutari.

Miller, S. Living with a disabled sibling – a review. *Paediatric Nursing,* **8(8),** 21–23.

Pennells, M. & Smith, S. (1995) *The Forgotten Mourners – Guidelines for Working with Bereaved Children.* London: Jessica Kingsley.

Smith, S. & Pennells, M. (eds.) (1995) *Interventions with Bereaved Children.* London: Jessica Kingsley.

Stewart, A. & Dent, A. (1994) *At a Loss – Bereavement Care when a Baby Dies.* London: Baillière Tindall.

Stewart, D., Stein, A., Forrest, G. & Clark, D. (1992) Psychosocial adjustment in siblings of children with chronic life-threatening illness: a research note. *Journal of Child Psychology and Psychiatry,* **33(4),** 779–784.

Children and parents in hospital

INTRODUCTION

There have been many changes in the ways children are cared for in hospitals, particularly since the early 1960s. Lansdown (1996), who has much experience of working with children in hospital, has researched the historical background. Lessons have been learnt from past experiences, when parents were only permitted to visit at specified times; children's wards today usually allow unrestricted access for parents. The National Association for the Welfare of Children in Hospital, now renamed Action for Sick Children, has fought hard for significant changes, encouraging parents to stay in hospital with their children. This has led to provision of accommodation on wards for a parent to sleep, usually in a bed beside the child. The Sick Children's Trust has built or adapted several houses, close to large hospitals, where families can stay while a child is in hospital. This is especially appreciated when a child is in hospital for long periods of time and the treatment is at a specialist centre far from home.

Family members are included in the care of a sick child; parents may negotiate their child's care plan and choose to perform certain elements of this in partnership with nursing staff. It sometimes takes a while to adapt to this 'parenting in public' (Darbyshire, 1994) and living in the ward, until roles are established and parents and nurses are sufficiently comfortable and confident. The fundamental fact remains for all parents that, whatever the reason for their child being in hospital, they are not there from choice, but because their child is sick. They are in a strange environment with people they do not know (at least at first) and away from home, family and friends. A range of emotions and feelings may surround them, as illustrated in Figure 12.1. These feelings and emotions may be powerful and have a significant impact on the way parents cope with the experience of being in hospital. If staff are aware of them and perhaps acknowledge

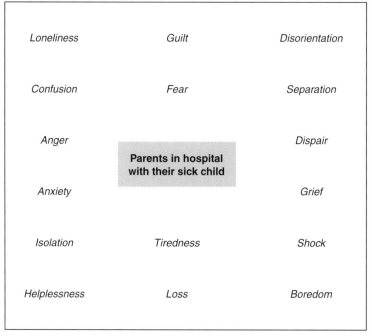

Figure 12.1 The range of emotions and feelings of parents in hospital with their children.

them with parents, it can be helpful in preventing some problems later, not the least of which is the 'labelling' of parents as being difficult.

PARENTS' DISORIENTATION AND CONFUSION

There are many reasons why parents may find it difficult to settle with their child in the ward or unit:

- concern for the child
- strange surroundings
- hospital routine
- lack of privacy
- threatening environment
- 'high-tech' equipment
- medical terminology
- the long hospital day, with associated boredom and isolation
- lack of sleep
- no usual chores, such as housework
- misunderstandings of information and instructions
- poor communication between parents and staff or among staff
- unpredictability leading to mental confusion
- separation from normal support of family and friends.

The staff can help parents considerably by giving good information, offering opportunities to talk, and keeping appointments and promises. This all helps in building trust.

CARING FOR PARENTS IN HOSPITAL

Caring for the parents of sick children is a question of supporting them during a period when they are unlikely to consider their own needs as a priority. Parents tell us frequently: 'I am all right, he's more important' and 'she needs me to be with her'. The state of the parent is directly proportional to the state of the child; when the child's condition improves, the parent feels better. It is not surprising that many mothers wait until they are at home after discharge before they allow themselves to relax.

Involvement in the care of a sick child is stressful for parents and some look to the nurses for support and care, although their primary patients are the children (Callery, 1997a). The health care team must recognise the family's strengths and individuality, and respect different methods of coping (Campbell, Kelly & Summersgill, 1993). A family's reactions to the crisis of a child in hospital will be unpredictable, as will the level of involvement in the child's care.

A study by Darbyshire (1995) found that parents had to perform the most delicate of social balancing acts. They had to be demonstrably caring, but not overly so, lest they be thought neurotic. They had to show great interest yet not take nurses' valued work away from them. They were to do whatever they would do at home yet also fit in with the hospital's policies and practices (Darbyshire, 1995)

Consideration for the welfare of the parents will include:

- somewhere to sleep – a bed, not a chair, beside the child, acknowledging the need for some privacy, e.g. by providing curtains around the bed if not in separate rooms
- bath or shower for parents to use
- facilities for washing, drying and ironing clothes
- sitting room for parents with facilities for making tea and coffee, a TV and a refrigerator
- telephones for outgoing and incoming calls (payphones)
- use of restaurants and other food outlets
- accommodation for mothers who are breastfeeding – privacy for feeding, pumps for expressing milk, sterile bottles and refrigerator and freezer for storage
- health of parents – may have, for example, a condition such as diabetes or asthma needing regular medication, or an

infection or tooth abscess that requires attention

- opportunities for parents to discuss their child's condition with the doctor, in a private setting if appropriate
- time to talk – to express fears and hopes, clear misunderstandings and make plans
- time to check on parents' understanding and coping, whether they are getting sufficient sleep, food and drinks, and how the rest of the family are managing at home.

Being in hospital can be expensive and most families notice how much extra money is needed to buy meals, newspapers and magazines, make telephone calls to family and friends and provide little treats for the children such as favourite drinks and sweets. Travelling to and from the hospital may be costly, especially if from a distance. Parents with low incomes who receive benefits may be eligible for some help with fares on admission and discharge. The bills at home still have to be paid and parents may lose income while they are in hospital with the child. Social workers will advise on any benefits to which parents may be entitled.

Callery (1997b) described the parents' financial commitment as open-ended and the burden of financial costs as inequitable, but the costs to parents of their involvement in the care of their hospitalised children have received little attention.

STRESS

The stresses of being in hospital only compound the underlying anxiety around the child's condition, which is stressful in itself. Parents under stress often say they do not 'function properly'. The coping mechanisms they would use normally may be inadequate, making them feel helpless and ineffective in making decisions, remembering facts or even noticing changes in the child's state. They may react somatically with headaches, nausea and sickness, constipation or diarrhoea.

Sources of stress are many, but the following are some that parents have raised:

- fear about procedures
- lack of information
- fear of the unknown
- fear of financial worries
- being in a new world, with new expectations
- being away from home
- loss of own identity

- no privacy
- no private possessions
- communication – lack of; cultural misunderstanding; language
- frustrations – waiting for test results; waiting to talk to a doctor
- making decisions
- being isolated
- partner stress
- guilt
- stressful environment
- lack of sleep
- boredom – 'nothing happening at weekends'
- resentment
- ward rounds
- medical students
- visitors
- telephone conversations in public.

CULTURAL CONSIDERATIONS

Some families have extra difficulties going to hospital, especially those from different backgrounds and cultures.

Language

Parents may not speak or understand English language and may not have relatives nearby who could interpret when doctors and nurses are giving important information. For some, English is not their first language and they might have difficulty understanding and discussing medical matters in anything but their native tongue, especially at a stressful time. Many hospitals have arrangements with outside interpreters who will help at short notice. Parents must be able to understand what is to be done for their child, and they should know to what they are consenting when signing a consent form.

Food

Certain foods are not permitted by some religions and it can offend parents if staff do not respect their views. Requirements must be written clearly in the child's care plan, and resident parents invited to bring in their own food if the hospital is unable to help.

Somewhere to pray

Most hospitals have a chapel, which although perhaps originally intended as a Christian facility can be used by members of other religions by agreement and arrangement.

ADMISSION TO A HOSPITAL WARD

Elective admission

This usually follows an outpatient appointment when the consultant has agreed to admit the child at a later date for surgery or treatment. This waiting time can be stressful, especially if the admission date is postponed because of illness or lack of available beds in hospital. A planned admission allows time to prepare a child for what she might experience, according to her age. Many hospitals send information booklets giving advice on what to take into hospital and how to tell the child what to expect. Some hospitals offer pre-admission visits for children, after school or on Saturday mornings. There are also a number of good story and picture books available which are helpful for children and parents before going into hospital.

Parents can become quite anxious about their child's admission and the child may sense their fears. Some parents can even feel more stressed about their child's admission to hospital than the child feels (Eiser, 1990); they may have their own memories of traumatic admissions as a child, or negative views. As Farrell (1995) wrote:

Hospitalisation of a child is likely to lead to emotional, social and environmental disturbance for the family and will affect the parental role. It is essential that health care staff build caring relationships with the sick child's parents.

Correct information is important for the parents; they need to understand what is to happen before they can explain it, in their own words, to the child. Lansdown (1996) suggested we should consider the possibility that knowledge in itself is not necessarily advantageous to children. Adults should think carefully about what a child needs to know, what is helpful and what might cause more anxiety and fear rather than help the child.

Emergency admissions

Most admissions of children to hospital are for medical or surgical emergencies, so there may not be time for preparation of the child or parents. The parents may be suffering not only from the stress of coping with the child's sudden illness and all the worries to do with that, but may be exhausted after a sleepless night caring for the sick child. The parents' priority is the urgent treatment of their child's condition, whether it is an asthma attack, appendicitis or a fractured limb, and they need to be reassured that the appropriate care is given.

Orientation on the ward

Whatever the reason for the child's admission, a member of the ward staff should show the parents around, giving clear guidance on issues such as where they can make hot drinks away from the risks of scalding active children, mealtimes for children, telephones, bathrooms, parents' room and other facilities. Children like to see the playroom and meet the play staff. The child's nurse will spend time with the parents, recording all the necessary information and discussing the child's care. The first impressions that parents gain from contact with hospital staff are vital for building a trusting relationship. Children also respond positively to a welcoming environment.

Adolescents in hospital

Patients in this age group would probably prefer to be admitted to a ward caring only for adolescents, but most hospitals do not offer this. Older teenagers might be admitted to an adult ward, and those under 16 to a children's ward. It is often possible to organise the beds so that the young people can be near others of a similar age. Some wards have prepared leaflets welcoming teenagers, giving them useful information suitable for their age. Considerations include watching television and videos after young children have gone to bed, help and advice for girls menstruating, privacy when being examined, information about their illness or operation, choice of menu other than young children's food and encouragement to share their worries and questions.

Adolescence is a difficult period in life for teenagers with no medical problems, so the physical and hormonal changes are often much more challenging for those with a chronic medical condition such as diabetes or cystic fibrosis, or those taking steroid or immunosuppression drugs. Clinic attendance can become poor or erratic; compliance with medical advice and prescribed self-care become inadequate and a source of stress between adolescent, parents and care-givers (Eiser, 1993).

As each adolescent is so different physically, psychologically and socially, depending on development, it is vital on admission that considerable time is given to the assessment process, so that factors which will affect the response to illness and hospitalisation can be identified, together with coping strategies that have been used successfully by the patient in the past to deal with stress (Kelly, 1991).

THE MULTIDISCIPLINARY TEAM

Children and parents expect to see doctors and nurses in hospital, but there are other important people too! Children's wards are likely to have nursery nurses and hospital play specialists, physiotherapists, psychologists, psychiatrists, dieticians, technicians from other departments, chaplains, ward clerks and cleaning staff. A friendly cleaner who talks to children and parents helps to make them welcome, and the physiotherapist can support parents in helping their child to cough, walk or do special exercises. Feeding a child is a basic essential for parents, but it can be frustrating and distressing when a sick child will not feed; they may feel rejected when a child vomits the food or milk they have given carefully. A dietician may become the person parents can trust to help them feed their child.

Psychologists offer help for behavioural problems, eating disorders, communication disorders, soiling, bed-wetting, constipation, anxiety management, depression, conversion (sometimes called hysterical) disorders, post-trauma and bereavement, and disclosure work in child protection situations. Paediatricians may ask them to see children whose physical symptoms are not explained organically or these who complain of a level or type of pain for which there does not seem to be an apparent cause. Play therapy may be helpful as a means of communication, allowing a child to express fears or tell a story though drawing or play. Children sometimes believe that their illness is somehow their own fault, and so need reassurance if this belief is expressed.

Psychiatrists would be asked to assess children for depression, psychoses and other psychiatric disorders, and also after suicide or overdose attempts. Some parents have strong fears or suspicions about someone with the title of psychologist or psychiatrist and are resistant to the suggestion that they might be helpful. Others welcome another 'specialist' opinion and want the best for their child. Either way, it is important that they are introduced as part of the team and part of the care of their child, in order to support the child and, in turn, them as parents.

School in hospital

Children have a right to receive suitable education while in hospital for a long time (Department of Health, 1996). This may mean going to hospital school or receiving help from visiting teachers. For many children, the teacher brings a touch of the 'normal' and an escape from illness. They may liaise with the children's schools, to provide teaching materials of the child's standard. Many teachers in hospitals have learnt much about children's medical conditions, but they need support and to be included in the caring team on the ward.

THE IMPORTANCE OF PLAY

When I was sick and lay a-bed,
I had two pillows at my head,
And all my toys beside me lay
To keep me happy all the day.
(R.L. Stevenson)

Play is always important for children – for fun, developing social skills, discovering and communicating. For children in hospital, play has extra values that are also supportive to them; Lansdown (1996) describes five particular functions:

- aiding normality
- the reduction of anxiety
- speeding recovery
- facilitating communication
- preparation for hospitalisation or for procedures.

Hospital play specialists are essential members of the team caring for children, providing them with normal toys, games and materials suitable for their age and ability, as well as for specialised play. Their skills are invaluable in helping children to understand procedures and treatments they need. Examples include injections and blood tests, insertion of feeding tubes and intravenous lines (particularly long lines or Hickman lines for chemotherapy), radiotherapy (making and wearing of masks), transplants, and, before going to theatre, dressing up in theatre hats and 'green pyjamas'. It is helpful for children and parents to be familiar with any unusual equipment in advance so that it does not increase their anxiety.

Children need to have a basic understanding of the body and its functions to enable them to make rational decisions regarding lifestyle and health (McEwing, 1996). Paediatric nurses have an essential role to play in the teaching and health education of sick children, as health education is inseparable from advocacy and children's rights (Gaudion, 1997). Some knowledge is necessary to enable children to understand why they are ill and what is going to happen to them. Anatomical dolls can help children to learn where the parts of their bodies are, their main functions and what is being done to make them better. It is often obvious from the relief on a parent's face that they are pleased to hear the information being given to the child, perhaps because they did not know how to explain it themselves or because they understand it better than when it was told to them.

Play specialists may work in conjunction with nurses, medical staff, counsellors and psychologists, helping individual children with particular difficulties. Learning relaxation and coping strategies can help children and teenagers to face frightening treatments and procedures. They may help children to talk about bad experiences and to work out their feelings through play. This is particularly relevant after a child has been involved in an accident or witnessed an event that is causing intrusive memories or nightmares (see Case Study 12.1).

CASE STUDY 12.1   Overcoming trauma through play

Lisa, aged 4 years, was a passenger in the car driven by her mother when it was in collision with a lorry. Her mother died in the car at the scene of the crash and Lisa was rescued and taken to hospital. She spent a few days in the children's intensive care unit and was then moved to a children's ward. As she became stronger, she began to play, assisted by a play specialist. On one occasion she was taking toys out of the playroom cupboard with her grandmother; Lisa picked up an ambulance and her grandmother immediately told her to put that back saying: 'Oh you don't want to play with that.' The play specialist noted this. Later on when the grandmother had gone, Lisa went to the cupboard again and took the ambulance. She told the play specialist that Mummy had gone in the ambulance, slammed the doors shut and pushed the ambulance away saying that Mummy was gone and was not coming back.

On another occasion Lisa picked a red car from the cupboard and her grandmother said she should play with a different coloured car, knowing that her mother's car in the accident was red. Lisa took a lorry and played with the two vehicles appearing to drive towards each other. She started to shout, 'The lorry's going out of control! There's going to be a crash!' and smashed the toys together. Then she picked them up, laid them carefully in the box and went back to her bed.

This young child needed to act out her traumatic memories of the accident in which her mother died, but her grandmother could not bear to hear it and tried to protect Lisa from thinking bad thoughts. Lisa's grandmother had lost her daughter and now felt responsible for protecting her child. The play specialist was able to allow Lisa to tell her story through play in a safe place. She later described Lisa's play to the grandmother, who was relieved that it had been discussed so that she did not have to be the first person to raise the subject.

CLINICAL PROCEDURES FOR CHILDREN

Many parents find it very difficult to be present while 'something nasty is being done' to their child, and yet they feel they must stay with them. They themselves may hate 'needles' and cannot really bear to watch the child have a blood test, much less be expected to hold them during the procedure. Some parents choose to go out and not be associated with it, returning to comfort and reassure the child afterwards. A study by Neill (1996) showed that parents preferred professionals to be responsible for their children's clinical care while they continued with the normal everyday care. We should not underestimate how much support the parents need during treatments and procedures for the child. They often say they wish they could have it done to them instead of the child.

There are ways of supporting parents when they feel unable to help their children, but it may take some planning, as for example in Case Study 12.2.

Preparation is important for both parents and children – talking through what will happen, how it might feel, how long it will take, and if there will be a bandage or plaster at the end. Despite the clearly demonstrated benefit of preparatory work with children and their parents, well-researched techniques are not yet widely incorporated into practice (While, 1992).

CASE STUDY 12.2   Supporting a distressed parent

Ricky was due to have his wound dressing changed for the first time since his operation to amputate his injured toes on one foot. His mother was frightened of seeing his foot which had been bandaged since the surgery. She tried hard not to cry in front of Ricky, but she was clearly very distressed and torn between staying outside the room and fulfilling her promise to stay with him.

Ricky was comfortable after his medication for pain relief and quite calm when he knew his mother was with him; she was relieved he was comfortable, but realised it was important to Ricky that she stayed as promised. A nurse prepared the treatment room and another stayed to support his mother. The plastic surgeon explained what he was going to do and how he expected the foot to look.

The surgeon and the nurse took up their positions by the trolley on one side of the bed and the other nurse sat with Ricky's mother on the opposite side. She sat with her back to Ricky's foot, so that he could see her face and hear her voice clearly even though he was rather sleepy from the medication.

> The surgeon and the nurse assisting him gave a commentary on how they were progressing and the nurse who was supporting his mother stayed right beside her, watching her closely as she frequently said she felt sick or faint. She needed encouragement to talk to Ricky and constant reassurance that she was 'doing well'. When the dressings were off and the wound cleaned, the surgeon described it to Ricky's mother in detail and said that he was pleased and hopeful that it was healing well. The supporting nurse encouraged his mother to ask questions and she gradually became more relaxed and relieved. She was finally able to take a look at the foot, again being well supported physically and emotionally. After that session, Ricky's mother went in with him for all his dressings and she felt pleased to have kept her promise to be with him.

SURGERY FOR CHILDREN

Parents and children may need considerable support before, during and after the operation. Adequate time is necessary for information and discussion before making decisions, as some parents are known to carry great burdens of responsibility and guilt for consenting to their child's operation. Parents say it makes the decision easier for them if the child is in agreement and takes a positive attitude to the treatment. A study by Alderson (1993) concluded that:

Decision making for children can be seen as an arena in which power shifts back and forth, as it is contested or shared between parents and professionals and, more recently, children. Professionals often have to decide when to treat parents as joint or rival or proxy clients, with or for the child, and how to balance the sometimes conflicting needs of the child-as-an-individual and the child-in-the-family.

Children who are of an age and understanding to make informed decisions about their treatment should be allowed to give or withhold consent. Health professionals must ensure that in the child's interest, simple but honest information has been understood and they know what to expect when they wake after an anaesthetic. It is not surprising that a 10-year-old refused to speak to her mother when, upon waking, she discovered a large abdominal wound – her mother had told her she was just going for a test.

Signing a consent form for a child's anaesthetic, operation or procedure may appear to be a simple formality, but for many parents it is extremely difficult. It is not uncommon for one parent to be unable to sign and to rely on the other one to do it. I have heard parents say that the responsibility was too great, that they would 'feel so guilty if anything went wrong, as it would be my fault'. Single parents may feel particularly vulnerable and need extra time to feel comfortable with making such decisions alone. Parents with poor English language may need interpreters to help them understand the information given and the wording on the form.

A parent is usually able to accompany a child to the anaesthetic room and be present until the child goes to sleep (Department of Health, 1996). The parent may need considerable support from the ward nurse on the way to theatre and in the waiting area, and particularly after leaving the child. Parents describe this moment of 'handing over' their child as heart-breaking. They feel guilty and responsible and yet completely helpless; most parents have tears or are close to tears. They usually appreciate being accompanied back to the ward, or wherever they are to wait during the operation, as it is easy to forget the way when distressed. Parents should be encouraged to take a break away from the ward and to have something to eat or drink during the wait. It gives them an opportunity to 'recharge their own batteries' before their child will need them later, and it also helps to fill the time that seems to pass so slowly.

It is common policy in many hospitals for parents to go to the recovery area with the ward nurse to collect the child, unless the child is returning to an intensive care unit. Parents like to know that they were there when their child woke up, and it is reassuring for children to hear a familiar voice through their drowsiness. The results of a research study by Brown (1995) showed that both parents and staff felt that great benefits resulted from an early parental presence in the recovery room. The parents felt they were involved in performing an active part in their child's care and that they were able to give them comfort. The children who woke in the recovery room were noticeably happier for being able to see a parent immediately, and the recovery staff benefited from the child's stay being less traumatic for the child.

I have mentioned already the importance of preparing parents for the child's condition and appearance after an operation. They build their own picture of what to expect and that is fundamental to their coping. It is therefore crucial to this coping that they are warned of any changes that may occur to their picture. A polaroid camera is very useful for taking instant photographs of the child to show the parents or siblings before they actually see her. Seeing a picture first allows them to express their shock or distress and perhaps cry safely with someone who can explain the details.

Sometimes the original plan, as discussed with the parents, has to be charged. An operation may take longer than was at first thought, the procedure may be more complicated and intravenous infusions and wound drains may be sited. There may have been problems with the anaesthetic or fluid balance and it may be felt prudent to observe the child in a high-dependency or intensive care unit instead of returning her to a ward postoperatively. This information should be given to the parents in a positive manner so that they understand that their child is being given the best possible care. Otherwise, they might panic, thinking that 'everything has gone wrong'.

CHILDREN IN AN INTENSIVE CARE UNIT

Admissions to a paediatric intensive care unit (PICU) may be elective, following major surgery such as cardiac surgery, neurosurgery, transplants, major surgery on young babies and procedures on children considered to have some anaesthetic or surgical risk. Babies born prematurely and needing respiratory assistance are usually admitted to a neonatal intensive care unit. When a PICU admission is planned, it is helpful for the parents and the child to visit the unit beforehand and be shown around. This gives them an opportunity to ask questions and to see the equipment that will be in use for the child postoperatively. In units which specialise in particular types of surgery, it may be part of the role of a specialist nurse to explain the postoperative care to families, and a visit to the PICU is an important part of this preparation. A study by Farrell and Frost (1992) indicated that parents have a strong need for information and relief of anxieties that they may have about their child's condition.

The majority of admissions to a PICU are for emergency treatment. This might be following accidental injury, sudden serious illness or worsening of an existing condition. A large number of children need intensive care following head or multiple injuries – mostly from traffic accidents, falls from windows, trees or horses, or blows to the head. Sadly, some injuries are from non-accidental causes. Other 'accidents' include burns, scalds and smoke inhalation. Any sort of accident creates deep feelings of guilt and blame in parents. Yet other reasons for admission include respiratory conditions, brain haemorrhage, sudden severe illness such as meningitis, septicaemia, peritonitis, ingestion of drugs and alcohol, near drowning and near-miss cot death.

All the families suffer from the shock of their child being admitted to a PICU; for most it is a new and unwelcome experience provoking great anxiety and uncertainty. The time spent developing the initial relationship with a family of a child on a PICU is important for informed and astute assessment of the needs of that family (Carter, 1993).

Transfer from another hospital

Children admitted to a PICU may previously have been taken to their local hospital, and then transferred after assessment, stabilisation or deterioration in their condition. This adds to the trauma for the family: finding the way to a hospital further away, being separated from the child during the 'blue light' ambulance journey, leaving other family members at home and having no time to prepare.

Some PICUs operate a retrieval service and send a team of doctor, nurse and equipment to the referring hospital on request. The child receives care from an experienced paediatric team who will transfer the child to the PICU. If this team appears friendly and efficient, the parents will start to build their trust in the new team; a mother explained how relieved she was when the team arrived and 'took over' the care of her child.

An information booklet for parents is helpful, giving directions to the hospital, telephone numbers and details about the PICU, car parking and facilities.

Family support

Some units have a member of staff designated for family support; PICUs are immensely stressful for patients, parents and staff and there is great potential benefit to all these people from having a trained counsellor in the PICU team (Cook, 1993). The results of a questionnaire in a neonatal intensive care unit (Curran, Brighton and Murphy, 1997) highlighted deficiencies in communication between staff and parents. They suggested that the provision of a dedicated unit psychologist or specially trained nurse would help to deal effectively with this and other issues.

A survey by Colville of all the PICUs in the UK indicated that the majority of units regularly involve psychological personnel in the care of their patients and families (Colville, 1998). In some units, the work of support and follow-up is in the job description of a specialist liaison nurse.

It is recognised that support for the family of the sick child should extend to the 'family' of the health care team caring for the child (British Paediatric Association, 1993):

There is a need for counselling or support staff specifically to provide for the psychological and emotional needs of the child and family. Such support staff should be available for all children in the intensive care unit.

It is important to recognise the needs of staff for support from each other, from managers, and, at times, from counselling or support staff.

Other parents with their children in the ward or unit may or may not be helpful and it is worth keeping an ear open for any comments from parents. Occasionally, one parent causes distress to another by relating her story with all the gory details or not respecting privacy or confidentiality. The 'know-all' person can easily upset another with totally incorrect information or gossip. Most parents in hospital with a sick child are very supportive of each other and share a friendly understanding of their feelings. When parents of critically ill children are aware that another child is dying or has died, they feel desperately vulnerable and frightened. They may have been told there is a chance that their child might die and this makes it real, reminding them that children can and do die in this place.

Supporting sick children in PICU

Many of the children and babies nursed in an intensive care unit will be sedated, and possibly ventilated, with continuous or regular analgesic and paralysing drugs. According to most children questioned after recovery, they do not remember this phase. When children are able to see, sit up and talk, care is needed to protect them from sights and sounds that might be frightening for them. A high-dependency area is usually quieter, away from the noises of monitors and other alarms, and is less frightening for children. It offers a useful intermediate phase before going to a ward. Some children might be aware of their surroundings and their state of health, so care is needed, especially during doctors' rounds, to ensure that any discussion or information not aimed at patients is out of earshot. Older children need to have explanations from medical and nursing staff about treatment and progress, because if they are not given the information they need to make sense of what is happening, they will imagine it.

The child's dignity should be respected at all times; parents appreciate attention to details like keeping some cover on – a sheet, duvet, pillowcase or some clothes. The cleanliness and comfort of the child are important for parents as well as children, and parents will usually like to help with this more normal task. Remember the favourite hair bands or special socks! A photograph of the child when well could be placed near the bed, to help them hold on to the image of their happy, well child, gaining inspiration for their continued hope for recovery. It may also be helpful for the staff to see what the child is really like, as an active child rather than a sick one attached to machines.

Parents should be encouraged to bring favourite toys, play tapes through headphones and read well-known stories, as well as stroking, holding, feeling and talking with the child when possible.

The needs of the parents

Woodfield (1997) stated that it should not be left to parents to request what they require, because even the most articulate parent, when placed in the stressful situation of having a critically ill child, may feel unable to express thoughts, feelings and needs. This emphasises yet again the importance of giving time and attention to the families. These families deserve to be cared for by medical and nursing staff with the necessary skills and experience, who are strong in their knowledge and ability and competent to discuss life-threatening situations with parents.

Parents whose children have left PICU have commented that it was very important for them to be able to put their trust in the team. A father said that their 'utter professionalism' had been essential and expected; there was no room for doubts in the team, as the parents had more than enough doubts in their own abilities at that time.

Good communication and honesty are essential for building trust. Parents who leave the room during a procedure need to be kept in touch with what is happening, so it is helpful if someone sees them with a progress report at intervals. This is especially important during resuscitation, when on-going information is crucial to their realistic understanding of the situation.

A separate quiet room is a valuable facility; this should not be the doctors' office or nurses' coffee room, and should be away from the clinical area with its telephones ringing and monitors alarming. Here, staff are able to interview relatives in private, giving them undivided attention and an opportunity to ask questions and express their feelings and emotions. When a child is critically ill or dying, a separate room offers the family members somewhere to be together, to talk, cry and make coffee or tea.

Some parents need permission to *not* stay with their child in the PICU, if they find the environment too stressful or cannot bear to see their child in that situation. They may have a quick look through the doorway and then stay in the parents' room. It helps them to keep in touch with the child's condition if nursing and medical staff can give them frequent bulletins; this also helps them to manage the guilt that they may feel for not being with the child. If treated gently and with understanding, most parents are able to increase the length of time they can spend in PICU after the first day or two.

Parents are often vulnerable and fearful in the PICU, and denial may be necessary to help them cope with the new situation. It is helpful to have supportive listeners, who will allow them to express their fears, and aim for a realistic acceptance of the situation.

A way of coping for some parents is to withdraw, not only physically, but also mentally and emotionally. They may fix on just one small detail, something that is safer and more manageable, such as the tape holding a tube in place. Some may immerse themselves in a book as a temporary escape from the unreal world around them. Parents who sit for hours by the bedside may become obsessive 'monitor-watchers' and call the nurse's attention to the slightest change. There is a potential danger that some will 'help' by turning off alarms as they have seen nurses do.

When a child is seriously ill or injured, many people other than the immediate family will be concerned. Staff in PICUs are used to talking to anxious grandparents, friends and teachers on the telephone. If a child is admitted with suspected meningitis, it is amazing how many people ring the hospital in a state of frenzy, desperate to find out if their child could catch it. Everyone needs to be reassured that the family general practitioner and public health departments are there to give advice.

Many tired parents cannot cope with speaking to endless well-meaning callers and are grateful if nurses give messages or progress reports agreed by them. Another source of stress for parents may be reporters from local newspapers who are trying to find out details, particularly following a road traffic accident or other public event. Some hospitals have a press officer who will deal with any press enquiries or issue condition reports on a patient. Staff should reassure parents that information regarding their child's name, address and condition will not be released without their knowledge.

Parents of a child needing intensive care may also need care and attention for themselves. This includes not only all the information to understand the care and treatment of their child, but the physical and emotional care of them. They may need reminding to eat and drink, and reassurance that a nurse will be with the child while they are away. Sometimes they need 'permission' from staff to go home to see their other children or to try to have a better night's sleep in their own bed. This must, of course, be underwritten with the promise to telephone them if there is any change in the child's condition. Many respond positively to the suggestion that they need to build up their strength while the child is ventilated, as they will need their energy later as the child wakes up.

The importance of involving parents in the care of each sick child is recognised, but little emphasis has been placed on the needs of the parents themselves (Farrell and Frost, 1992). The results of a questionnaire to parents of children in an intensive care unit (Farrell and Frost, 1992) showed that information about the child was the most important factor. Of highest importance, by 96% of respondents, was 'to know what is wrong with my child', 'to be informed of any changes in my child's condition' and 'to have my questions answered honestly'. Other needs which scored highly included:

- to know the expected outcome
- to have explanations in understandable terms
- to know what treatment the child is receiving
- to talk with the doctor and the nurse
- to know the nurses are giving the best care possible
- to have a nurse at the bedside
- to be allowed to call the unit at any time
- to have the equipment explained
- to be told there is hope.

Transfer from PICU to the ward

Many parents will celebrate moving out of the PICU as official recognition that their child is 'getting better', 'over the worst' or 'a step nearer going home'. But other parents may feel very anxious at leaving the unit that 'saved their child's life', where there was a nurse with the child day and night and frequent visits from a doctor. However much they hated being in there with their child, feeling helpless, frightened and confused, they had trusted the staff and felt secure.

Moving to a ward is a big step for some parents and care is needed to prepare them beforehand, giving some warning of plans and perhaps taking them to see where the child will be. A detailed medical and nursing 'handover' is essential and families usually appreciate visits from familiar PICU staff, helping to ease the change. It is easy to understand why some parents comment that the care is not as good as PICU when they first go to a ward; they have become accustomed to one-to-one care and it can be rather different, but still appropriate, on a busy ward.

The PICU experience is traumatic and exhausting for most parents. Some have found it helpful to sit down and talk through what it was really like for them, a sort of 'debriefing' before moving on. It should be recognised that some families may take several weeks, or even months, to recover from the distressing time while a child was critically ill, displaying their own symptoms of post-traumatic stress. Writing about personal feelings and thoughts, perhaps keeping a diary, is therapeutic for some parents with children in a PICU or on a ward. If the child's progress is slow, as is often the case with head-injured children, it can be reassuring to look back and be reminded what it was like last week or last month, and realise just how much improvement there has been.

Children may be transferred from a PICU, a high-dependency unit or a ward at a regional centre to complete their recovery at their local hospital. It may be difficult for the parents to leave a now familiar unit in which they have established trust, even though it suits the family to be nearer home. Effective liaison between medical and nursing staff and other professionals such as physiotherapists and dieticians will help to reassure parents that the care will continue.

GOING HOME

Whatever the reason for a child's stay in hospital, going home to familiar toys, pets, bedroom and family is always special for the child. Most parents are also happy to be returning to some family normality. There may, however, be some nervous hesitation by parents, perhaps concerns about their ability to cope with new medications or treatments. In a study by Bailey and Caldwell (1997), a small proportion of parents wanted more information or discussion about the planned time of discharge. This is an ongoing problem with acute paediatric admissions, because of the unpredictable improvement rate of the child's condition and because paediatricians are not constantly available on the wards. When children have been critically ill or suffered accidental injury, their parents may lose confidence and need frequent reassurance and support from the hospital and community health professionals.

In some situations, parents may be given open access to the ward if they become concerned about their child's condition. This may apply to a child with a chronic, life-threatening or terminal illness and helps parents to feel reassured that they will be able to get help for the child as and when it is needed. A book with these children's details in it, kept on the ward, makes the sudden appearance of a child in the accident and emergency department or on the ward easier for the family and the on-call staff who may not know the child.

CONCLUSION

Time spent in hospital is a very individual experience, different for each parent of each child and from one child to another. It may be traumatic, exhausting, worrying or frightening and yet a family may be grateful, appreciative and happy. The memories will probably be both good and bad, and the scars of the parents may be deeper than the child's; the child may bear the physical effects, but the parents certainly carry the emotional burden. Many professionals are involved when a child is in hospital; good communication and teamwork are essential, and it is important for all concerned to remember that the parents are also part of the team caring for their child.

REFERENCES

Alderson, P. (1993) *Children's Consent to Surgery*. Buckingham: Open University Press.

Bailey, R. & Caldwell, C. (1997) Preparing parents for going home. *Paediatric Nursing*, 9(4), 15–17.

British Paediatric Association (1993) *The Care of Critically Ill Children*, p 49. London: BPA (now Royal College of Paediatrics and Child Health).

Brown, V. (1995) Parents in recovery: parental and staff attitudes. *Paediatric Nursing*, 7(7), 17–19.

Callery, P. (1997a) Caring for parents of hospitalized children: a hidden area of nursing work. *Journal of Advanced Nursing*, 26(5), 992–998.

Callery, P. (1997b) Paying to participate: financial, social and personal costs to parents of involvement in their child's care in hospital. *Journal of Advanced Nursing*, 25(4), 746–752.

Campbell, S., Kelly, P. & Summersgill, P. (1993) Putting the family first: interpreting a framework for family centred care. *Child Health*, 1(2), 59–63.

Carter, B. (ed.) (1993) *Manual of Paediatric Intensive Care Nursing*. London: Chapman and Hall.

Colville, G. (1998) Psychosocial support on the paediatric intensive care unit: a UK survey. *Care of the Critically Ill*, 14(1), 25–28.

Cook, P. (1993) The value of family counselling in paediatric intensive care. Abstracts from The Paediatric Intensive Care Society Spring Meeting, March 1993. *Care of the Critically Ill*, 9(4), 179.

Curran, A., Brighton, J. & Murphy, V. (1997) Psychoemotional care of parents of children in a Neonatal Intensive Care Unit: results of a questionnaire. *Journal of Neonatal Nursing*, 3(1), 25–29.

Darbyshire, P. (1994) *Living with a Sick Child in Hospital; the Experiences of Parents and Nurses*. London: Chapman and Hall.

Darbyshire, P. (1995) Family-centred care within contemporary British paediatric nursing. *British Journal of Nursing*, 4(1), 31–33.

Department of Health (1996) *The Patient's Charter – Services for Children and Young People*. London: HMSO.

Eiser, C. (1990) *Chronic Childhood Disease – an Introduction to Psychological Theory and Research*. Cambridge: Cambridge University Press.

Eiser, C. (1993) How teenagers cope with chronic illness and compliance. *Maternal and Child Health*, May, 148–150.

Farrell, M. (1995) The effect of a child's hospitalisation on the parental role. *Professional Nurse*, **10(9)**, 561–563.

Farrell, M. & Frost, C. (1992) The most important needs of parents of critically ill children: parents' perceptions. *Intensive and Critical Care Nursing*, **8**, 130–139.

Gaudion, C. (1997) Children's knowledge of their internal anatomy. *Paediatric Nursing*, **9(5)**, 14–17.

Kelly, J. (1991) Caring for adolescents. *Professional Nurse*, **6(9)**, 498–502.

Lansdown, R. (1996). *Children in Hospital – a Guide for Family and Carers*. Oxford: Oxford University Press.

McEwing, G. (1996) Children's understanding of their internal body parts. *British Journal of Nursing*, **5(7)**, 423–429.

Neill, S. J. (1996) Parent participation: literature review and methodology. *British Journal of Nursing*, **5**, 34–40.

Stevenson, R. L. (1994) The land of counterpane. In *A Child's Garden of Verses*. Ware: Wordsworth Editions.

While, A. E. (1992) The contribution of nurses to children's well-being in hospital: a selective review of the literature. *Journal of Clinical Nursing*, **1(3)**, 117–121.

Woodfield, T. (1997) Parents of critically ill children: do we meet their needs? *Paediatric Nursing*, **9(8)**, 22–23.

FURTHER READING

Action for Sick Children (1992) *Ten Targets for the 1990s*. London: Action for Sick Children.

Blair, K. (1995) Facilities for parents. *Paediatric Nursing*, **7(4)**, 18–21.

British Association for Counselling – Counselling in Medical Settings Division (1995) *Guidelines for staff employed to counsel in hospital and health care settings*. BAC, Rugby.

Davis, H. (1993) *Counselling Parents of Children with Chronic Illness or Disability*. Leicester: BPS Books.

Department of Health (1991) *The Welfare of Children and Young People in Hospital*. London: HMSO.

Douglas, J. (1993) *Psychology and Nursing Children*. Leicester: BPS Books.

East, P. (1995) *Counselling in Medical Settings*. Buckingham: Open University Press.

Edwards, M. and Davis, H. (1997) *Counselling Children with Chronic Medical Conditions*. Leicester: BPS Books.

Faulkner, A. (1992) *Effective Interaction with Patients*. Edinburgh: Churchill Livingstone.

Weller, B. (1980) *Helping Sick Children Play*. London: Baillière Tindall.

Family support in the community

INTRODUCTION

It is generally acknowledged that the best place to care for children is at home with their families. One of the '10 targets for the 1990s' set by Action for Sick Children (1992) is: 'Whenever possible sick children should be cared for at home, unless the care they require can only be provided in hospital.'

Sadly, not all children are able to live full and active lives; many are born with, or subsequently develop, health problems, and others have disabilities following illness and injury. Some families have to face an uncertain future with children suffering from life-threatening or life-limiting illnesses; their lives can never be 'normal', however hard they try.

Hospital-at-home is a relatively new concept, but is being increasingly embraced with the move towards care in the community (Bishop, Anderson & McCulloch, 1994). There are many children who are able to remain at home, rather than in hospital, including some children needing nursing and management of traction (Clayton, 1997). Home support not only benefits families in psychological terms, but may help to reduce complications (Cuttell *et al.*, 1996).

The services available to help these families vary between districts, but will probably include acute and primary health care services, social services, education services, voluntary organisations and parents' groups. This chapter considers some of the issues relating to families and ways of meeting their needs.

SUPPORT NEEDS OF FAMILIES WITH A SICK CHILD AT HOME

These needs can be grouped under the following headings (Maynard *et al.*, 1996):

- informational
- practical

- social
- emotional
- educational
- financial.

Some families are unable to manage without considerable help, because of family circumstances or the demands of the child's care. A multidisciplinary and multi-agency teamwork approach may be necessary in order to ensure the family is offered the help needed, without duplicating and wasting resources.

Information

Parents need to be informed about the child's medical condition, treatment and prognosis, and what it means in relation to the family life. Telling parents that their child has a life-threatening illness may not be easy for the doctor, but how this is done could be significant to the family's subsequent coping. A study by Woolley *et al.* (1989) highlighted the value of open, sympathetic, direct and uninterrupted discussion of the diagnosis in private, giving sufficient time for parents to take the news in and for doctors to repeat and clarify information: 'The doctor's ability to accept and understand the parents' grief was important in establishing trust and shaping the future relationship' (Woolley *et al.*, 1989). The family GP and hospital doctors are vital for continuing help in this field of support.

Another good source of information might be a support group for the child's particular condition. The *Contact-a-Family Directory* (Contact-a-Family, 1998) lists over 200 specific conditions and rare syndromes in children, giving medical descriptions of the conditions and the support groups and contacts willing to help. It also includes notes on inheritance patterns and prenatal diagnoses, and a list of regional genetics centres and helpful organisations.

Many support groups issue information leaflets about the conditions and their complications. Some publish newsletters and have local groups for support and fundraising. It is not only being given information that parents find helpful, but also discussing and sharing it with others who understand. These people might be health professionals or other parents who have a child with similar problems. Many parents say they need to have all the available information in order to understand the difficulties, know the possible options and be able to make choices for their child and for the family. Information leaflets can be given to relations and friends, helping parents to explain the illness and its related problems.

Information about benefits, allowances, or equipment may be relevant and help is available through the social services and advice centres. The local community health council may hold a database of all available sources of help. Some teams, such as area children's disability teams, have produced booklets containing the addresses and telephone numbers of all the organisations and agencies that might be helpful for parents of children with special needs of any kind. This is very useful for families who do not know what help and advice are available, or how to find it.

Practical help

The Patient's Charter (Department of Health, 1996) states that parents can expect to care for their child at home whenever possible and can expect appropriate support to do this. Parents need advice and guidance from various professionals in order to learn what is available to help them. Most parents would not know where to begin if they have not had any previous experience. Good liaison between the hospital and the community paediatric nursing team is probably the first step; they are often the key professionals in organising support.

Some neonatal units offer a community neonatal nursing service. This enables parents to take home premature babies or those needing some nursing care, including babies dependent on oxygen therapy. Specialist nurses supervise the care of these children and babies, giving parents the help and support they need. It is helpful, not only for the families but also for the nurses' own confidence and survival, if these professionals have some training in counselling skills and bereavement care.

The community nurses help parents to manage procedures that could be performed at home. These might include feeding through a nasogastric or gastrostomy tube, caring for a tracheostomy, giving oxygen, administering medication for seizures, caring for indwelling lines such as a Portcath or Hickman lines and giving intravenous medication or total parental nutrition. Sidey and Torbet (1995) reported that when well managed by children's nurses, dieticians and families, enteral feeding can be useful with little disruption to a normal family-centred lifestyle.

Medical equipment may be required as part of the child's care, either routinely or in an emergency. It is possible to have certain items on loan from a hospital, a community nurses' supply or the manufacturer. These might include oxygen cylinders, portable suction machines, wheelchairs, hoists, ramps and many more. Some disposable items are available on prescription or from the hospital. Social services, occupational therapists and physiotherapists may make assessments of the child and family needs. The local pharmacist can provide good support, ensuring the child's supplies of medicines and helping parents to understand their uses.

Parents need to be given telephone numbers of people they can call when they have questions or problems. These may be 'key workers', a 'link person' or any of the professionals in the multidisciplinary team.

Social support

Caring for a sick child at home is hard work, physically and emotionally, whether it is short-term, long-term or terminal care. Some parents are reluctant to have help in the house, let alone have someone else care for their child. It is perhaps understandable that parents do not want to leave a very sick or dying child with someone outside the family, but other children in the family have their needs, and the couple's relationship benefits from some time together.

Respite care may be available in different ways. Some areas operate a service that gives parents a few hours a week of 'time off'. A children's nurse goes to the home, allowing parents time for shopping, to spend with the other children, an evening out or some undisturbed sleep. Whilst most parents would not wish for a hectic social life when they have to care for their child, it is important to remember that they do have a life of their own. A mother once said to me: 'I would like people to sometimes think of me by *my* name and not only to be known as Jo's mother. I would like to be asked how *I* am, not always "how is Jo?".'

Hospices for children

There are a number of hospices for children around the country, which offer excellent respite care for families. The main themes (Maynard *et al.*, 1996) addressed by the paediatric hospice philosophy are:

- the provision of flexible care and support for the whole family
- help with symptom control and the physical problems of daily living
- continuity of support after a child's death.

Farrell (1996) concluded that the real benefit of a children's hospice lies in the fact it provides families of very sick children with another choice at a time when their ability to exercise choice or control over the painful situation in which they find themselves is severely limited. Sister Francis Dominica founded the first hospice for children in Britain, Helen House in Oxford, which opened in 1982. She believes hospice is a philosophy rather than a facility, a whole approach rather than an in-patient unit (Dominica, 1990):

This approach is practised wherever there is a child who suffers from an illness which is a threat to survival, whether the child is at home, in hospital, in residential care, in school, or in a hospice building.

Emotional support

Parents with a sick child, or one with special needs or a disability, grieve for the 'normal' child they no longer have or never had. With this grief comes a range of strong feelings and emotions which add to the physical tiredness of caring. Extended family and friends may offer good support and share the feelings, but it may be more helpful to talk to someone outside the family. Psychological support might be available from a counsellor at the health centre, hospital, family consultation clinic, social services or church, or from an independent counsellor.

Eiser (1990) emphasised the need to understand how ordinary families deal with specific crises that arise; families and children dealing with chronic disease are not seen as deviant, but as ordinary people in exceptional circumstances. 'Coming to terms' with a child's condition, treatment and prognosis may not be easy and takes time.

Psychologists are part of the team caring for children. They are skilled at assessing the psychological factors in children's illness or disability, especially if the symptoms are not fully explained physically. They help children to discuss or express through play their worries, fears and difficulties at home or school. Psychologists help children to manage depression and anxiety, behavioural skills, problem-solving and communication disorders.

Family therapy might be helpful for the family of a child with a chronic problem. The siblings may be feeling left out and unimportant, and parents will not be used to their altered behaviour. All family members may become confused, angry and frightened, making it more difficult to cope with life. The therapist facilitates sessions and encourages all members to speak openly in front of the others. In this way, misconceptions can be aired and discussions entered into in order to help family members work through the problems highlighted.

Many couples find that their relationship suffers under the strain of being unable to give each other time and attention. Misunderstandings and poor communication lead easily to arguments, making an already difficult situation worse, at a time when they need to support both themselves and the partnership. Counselling for couples helps many to work out some of these difficulties and to cope better with their strained relationship.

Spiritual support may or may not be part of a family's support system when a child is sick. Parents may be angry with God that He should allow this to happen to their child and their family; alternatively, they might find great comfort in their faith. Local clergy and ministers of all faiths are available to help during this confusing and sometimes lonely spell, when parents, in particular, need all the strength they can gather.

Educational support

Education plays a large and important role in a child's life, whether the child is fit and well or has minor or major problems. Children who are able to get to school benefit from the more normal routine of the school day and the security of being among familiar friends and teachers. Teachers may not understand the implications of a child's life-threatening condition, and unless they have had previous experience or made special enquiries, they may not feel able to help the child and family talk about the problems. When a child has been absent from school for a period of illness or treatment, it is important for teachers to welcome the child back gently, perhaps preparing the child's peers beforehand.

Many children who have medical conditions and health problems have been assessed by the local education authority and have written statements of special education needs. They may receive extra help from classroom assistants or spend part of the school day in a group for children with special needs. Some children have a home teacher who gives a few hours of individual teaching per week, either instead of or in conjunction with some school attendance.

A working party on behalf of the Royal College of Paediatrics and Child Health (1997) reported that the needs met under the Education Act 1993 are:

- the need for children's special educational needs to be identified as early as possible

- the need for parents to be involved in the provision of resources to help their child
- the need for children with special needs and their parents to be provided with a co-ordinated provision from all the services concerned.

Clearly, there must be discussion between parents and all professionals involved in a child's care to establish what help would be appropriate and what might be available. Depending on the area where a family lives, special schools for deaf, blind or physically handicapped children may be suitable. The local authority usually provides transport, whether the school is nearby or outside the area. Some of these schools have residential accommodation with trained children's nurses in attendance. This is the only feasible option for some parents of severely handicapped children, who could not manage to care for the child at home, except for short periods with help. They may feel very guilty about 'abandoning' their child and be devastated if the child dies when they are not with them. Staff at the school should be well supported following attempted resuscitation and deaths, which do happen at these special schools.

Day schools for children with special needs care for children with many different problems. Some children need regular medication, including for the control of seizures, and teachers and other staff have to feel competent and confident at giving the treatment. Parents need to feel they can trust the staff in their absence.

There are many children in mainstream school who need to take medication regularly, and others who must have medicines available for emergencies. A small number of children suffer from severe allergic reactions and may go into anaphylactic shock, requiring an immediate injection of adrenalin. School teachers can be anxious about giving this, understandably, and appropriate education must be given. A plan of action in case of emergency should be written in collaboration with the community paediatrician, the school and the parents.

There are many children with chronic illness and disabilities and with life-threatening conditions who attend normal school, and they need to be supported fully. The teaching staff may appreciate support from the hospital, community nurses and school nurses and help to understand a child's condition and treatment. An example of good liaison in support of children is the work done by some regional centres for paediatric oncology. The paediatric community nurses and specialist nurses offer information and advice about cancer and leukaemia to the schools of their patients. This helps the teachers to learn about the illness and the treatments and how that may affect the child's schooling. It helps them to support the child in school and also to help the other children, who may want to know, for example, why a child wears a hat in school (because his hair has fallen out during chemotherapy).

Children returning to school after a period away are likely to experience some difficulties. They 'lose their place' in various ways: they miss parts of the school curriculum so that the others in the class have moved on to new work; former friends may have made friends with other children and the returning child feels left out; the child may feel some shame at not being 'right', i.e. not like the rest of the peer group. Education is therefore important for all children, whatever the circumstances. The normalisation of a sick child's life is a good aim, even for a dying child.

Financial support

Most families with a sick child experience some financial hardship; even parents of a child who is sick for only a short time notice difficulties. One parent is usually unable to work as a result of having to care for the child, and sometimes the other parent stays at home to look after siblings, especially if frequent hospital visits or admissions are necessary. Single parents usually have less choice and may rely on benefits for income.

The family may face extra bills for heating, hot water, washing, telephones, special diet foods, clothing, transport to hospital appointments, babysitting and help at home. Advice centres and social services advise people about their entitlement to benefits and special payments. Some charities are able to offer some financial support for certain situations, but most families have some employment and financial difficulties.

CHILD PROTECTION ISSUES

Most areas have specific guidelines for all staff working with children, whether in hospitals, clinics, residential homes or schools. If a child is admitted to hospital and there is any suspicion of non-accidental injury, or sexual, emotional or physical abuse, the procedure must be followed. Good teamwork is important, especially between the hospital and the area social work team who are responsible for making the investigations. Other professionals involved will probably include the GP, health visitor, schoolteacher and the police.

These matters are not easy. It is essential for the protection of staff, as well as the child, to follow the statutory procedures. Good support for staff in all disciplines is also important, both for achieving what is best for the child and for their own emotional needs.

CONCLUSION

The key word, once again, is teamwork, with all disciplines and agencies working together for the good of the child and family. The Royal College of Nursing (1993):

...believes passionately that severely ill children have the right to be nursed at home as appropriate. What is needed is that both purchasers and those within provider units, including GP practices, recognise that paediatric community nursing services are essential services.

Another document (Department of Health, 1991) states: 'children are admitted to hospital only if the care they require cannot be as well provided at home, in a day clinic, or on a day basis in hospital'.

All children and their families live in 'the community', which is a word in common use and with many meanings, but which I understand to mean 'not in hospital'! It is where people live, work and play, according to their circumstances. There are many professionals working in the community to help sick children and their families. What they do and how to find them are not always obvious; making a start by *asking someone* will probably lead to more information and help. A good place to start is usually the GP surgery or health centre.

Faulkener, Peace and O'Keefe (1995) noted that GPs themselves emphasise the value of their role continuing through all stages of the child's illness, from diagnosis through treatment. They identified the GP's role in caring for the whole family, in three areas:

• knowledge and awareness of the individual family dynamics
• availability to offer support with living with uncertainty
• mobilisation of local resources to enable easier adjustment to 'normal' life within the community.

Support in the community is not solely directed at the child in isolation, but at each of the family members and their individual and collective needs. Professionals should provide support individually but also collectively, as a team. They also need to be well supported professionally and with time and resources. Casey's (1988) partnership model of care for children emphasises that 'children are best cared for by their family with varying degrees of assistance from members of a suitably qualified healthcare team whenever necessary'. Gould (1996) argued that a partnership with parents and family is more easily facilitated at home, where the environment is more comfortable and less threatening or frightening for the child and the parents. However, community support is not only required in the family home, but also at school, especially for children with special needs, and in nursery and child care facilities. It could involve many people from different disciplines. The key once again is good communication, teamwork and mutual support for the family in partnership with health care professionals.

REFERENCES

Action for Sick Children (1992) *Ten Targets for the 1990s*. London: Action for Sick Children.

Bishop, J., Anderson, A. & McCulloch, J. (1994) Hospital at home: a critical analysis. *Paediatric Nursing*, **6(6)**, 12–15.

Casey, A. (1988) A partnership with child and family. *Senior Nurse*, **8(4)**, 8–9.

Clayton, M. (1997) Traction at home: the Doncaster approach. *Paediatric Nursing*, **9(2)**, 21–23.

Contact-a-Family (1998) *Directory of Specific Conditions and Rare Syndromes in Children with their Family Support Networks*, 2nd edn (with six-monthly updates). London: Contact-a-Family.

Cuttell, K., Gartland, C., Argles, J. & Watson, A. (1996) Evaluation of a home care renal nursing service. *Paediatric Nursing*, **8(2)**, 16–18.

Department of Health (1991) *Welfare of Children and Young People in Hospital*. London: HMSO.

Department of Health (1996) *The Patient's Charter – Services for Children and Young People*. London: HMSO.

Dominica, Sister Frances (1990) Hospices: a philosophy of care. In *Listen, My Child has a Lot of Living to Do – Caring for Children with Life-threatening Conditions*, ed. Baum, J.D., Sister Francis Dominica & Woodward, R.N. Oxford: Oxford University Press.

Eiser, C. (1990) Psychological effects of chronic disease. *Journal of Child Psychology and Psychiatry*, **31**, 85–98.

Farrell, M. (1996) The role of a children's hospice. *Paediatric Nursing*, **8(4)**, 6–8.

Faulkener, A., Peace, G. & O'Keeffe, C. (1995) *When a Child has Cancer*. London: Chapman and Hall.

Gould, C. (1996) Multiple partnerships in the community. *Paediatric Nursing*, **8(8)**, 27–31.

Maynard, L., Barclay, S., Palmer, R., Todd, C. & Vickers, D. (1996) *Families in Need – the Needs of Families Caring for Children with Life-threatening Illnesses in Cambridge Health District*. Cambridge: Lifespan Healthcare NHS Trust.

Royal College of Nursing (1993) *Buying Paediatric Community Nursing*. London: RCN.

Royal College of Paediatrics and Child Health (1997) *The Essentials of Effective Community Health Services for Children and Young People – Report of a Working Party.* London: RCPCH.

Sidey, A. & Torbet, S. (1995) Enteral feeding in community settings. *Paediatric Nursing,* **7(6),** 21–23.

Woolley, H., Stein, A., Forrest, G.C. & Baum, J.D. (1989) Imparting the diagnosis of life threatening illness in children. *British Medical Journal,* **298,** 1623–1626.

FURTHER READING

Hughes, J. (1997) Reflections on a community children's nursing service. *Paediatric Nursing,* **9(4),** 21–23.

Whiting, M. (1997) Community children's nursing: a bright future? *Paediatric Nursing,* **9(4),** 6–9.

The death of a child

14

INTRODUCTION

The death of a child is always difficult for the family to bear, but also for those who witness their distress. There is something unjust and untimely about cutting short a young life. Parents do not expect to outlive their children, and often comment that they expected their child to bury them, not the other way around.

A death results not only in the loss of a precious child, but also in the loss of the family's hopes and aspirations for that child, the plans and imaginations for the life ahead. There is a sense of loss of the parents' future; grandparents feel this particularly, as they will not be handing on through the generations. Many expectations for the future will never be fulfilled – they will not see that child grow up, go to school, become independent and go to work, be married, have children (their grandchildren) and perhaps care for them in their old age.

Many good books and articles have been written about caring for dying children (e.g. Baum *et al.*, 1991; Bluebond-Langner, 1978; Goldman, 1994; Hill, 1994; Judd, 1995; Stewart and Dent, 1994; Wilkinson, 1991). Bereaved parents have written of their experiences surrounding the death of their child and how they struggled with their grief afterwards (e.g. Hill, 1989; Kushner, 1981; Spufford, 1989; Stuart and Totterdell, 1990). Other bereaved parents often find help and comfort in reading what parents have said, and those who write down their memories and thoughts usually find it therapeutic.

FAMILY-CENTRED CARE OF A DYING CHILD

In all aspects of caring for sick children, we aim to care for the whole family, but it seems especially important to involve as many family members as appropriate when a child is dying. The care and support they receive at this time plays a vital role in how they cope, not only with the actual death, but also during the weeks and months ahead.

Mothers and fathers

Parents may feel guilty that they are not able to make their child better. This sense of guilt is often particularly strong if the child had a sudden illness or was badly injured in an accident. One parent may blame the other, even if it is not expressed.

Many parents of dying children have separated, often adding to the mixed emotions, and some have new partners. This can cause arguments about who should be with the child and who makes decisions for the child. There may be feelings of guilt and blame. The natural mother and father would normally be regarded as the child's closest relatives but situations will vary. Professionals sometimes have to act in the child's best interest to prevent unpleasant behaviour amongst relatives, and may need to restrict the numbers of visitors and the visiting times. Hospital staff need to make it quite clear that they are there to nurse the sick child and not to get involved with family disputes. A plan could be drawn up, listing who may visit and when.

Even the strongest relationships come under great pressure during such an emotional time as this. A couple may find it really difficult to share their thoughts and feelings with each other and may need some help in acknowledging that they are each dealing with the situation in rather different ways. It is not unusual for one parent to try to 'be strong' for the other, even to the extent of denying the truth of what is happening. The father may be trying to be realistic, but may not feel it is right to destroy the optimism of his partner, the result being that neither is able to share fears and concerns with the other (see Case Study 14.1).

CASE STUDY 14.1 *'Coping' can harm communication*

The doctors had told Tina and Darren that their baby boy could not survive more than a few days longer. Both of the young parents tried hard to be cheerful for each other and avoided talking about the fact that the baby would die soon. When Tina went out of the room, Darren would speak to the nurse and say that he was worried about her. He did not know how she would cope with this dreadful time ahead.

When Darren went out, Tina would tell the nurse that she was very worried about Darren and she did not know how he was going to cope. When they were together, the nurse acknowledged that this was a difficult time for both of them and that it was probably hard for them to talk to each other because each of them was trying to be strong for the other. They admitted that this was true. They were both finding it impossible to tell their parents the truth of the situation, when they were trying to be so positive for Tina and Darren. Nobody in the family could bear to be honest, and the denial was becoming a barrier between Tina and Darren at the time when they needed to be close.

They seemed pleased when the nurse asked if they would like the hospital chaplain to visit them. The baby was to have been christened soon in their village church and they discussed this with the chaplain. A baptism was planned for a time when all their family and friends could be present.

The baby was dressed in new clothes and the small room was filled with visitors and nurses. The chaplain spoke about his short life, which had been normal until a few days before, and said that his family had now grown to include the doctors and nurse who were caring for him. The chaplain prayed for the baby, that God would keep him safe on his journey from this life, for his family who were grieving and for the hospital staff who had tried so hard to make him better. Most people were crying and holding each other during the short ceremony.

Afterwards, Darren explained how important the christening service had been; he called it a watershed and said they would be 'all right' now. It had been an acknowledgement of the truth and a sharing for everyone there. Darren and Tina faced their baby's death with dignity and love for him and for each other.

If the child has a single parent, there are extra considerations, among which is the reason for the parent being single. A recent divorce or death of a partner will be a loss to consider in the context of another imminent loss. The parent may feel desperately alone and in need of extra support from the grandparents or other friends and relations.

Brothers and sisters (see also Ch. 11)

Siblings should not be left out when one of them is very sick and dying. They need someone to support them if their parents are not able to give them the time and attention they need. The extent of their involvement will depend on their age and family circumstances. If the sick child is in hospital, it may not be easy to visit frequently, whereas at home the siblings may be able to help more.

Children in the same family will have their own feelings about what is happening. They may fear that the same terrible fate awaits them, that it was their fault or that they might have been able to prevent it happening. This is particularly significant if they witnessed the accident.

Grandparents

Grandparents often feel strong emotions when a grandchild is going to die, sometimes even suggesting that they are the ones who should be dying. They go back to being parents again, caring for their own child who is hurting with the pain of losing a child. They feel helpless, not knowing what they can do to help yet being careful not to interfere. Time for them to talk with those caring for the family is usually helpful. It gives them an opportunity to ask their own questions about the child's condition instead of always asking the parents, and the person giving the information may guide them in ways to help. If they have a good relationship with the family, grandparents have a valuable role in helping with other children and looking after their home.

It is interesting to note how many grandmothers facing the death of a grandchild will reflect on their own past history. When given the opportunity to talk with a nurse, chaplain or counsellor, they talk about a miscarriage, stillbirth or death of a baby or child that happened a generation ago, but which they may not yet have grieved for. They may not have been given the chance to see the dead body, attend a funeral or know what happened to the body. At least one grandmother I knew wanted to help wash and dress her daughter's baby after she died. She knew how important this would be for her daughter as she had not been able to do it for her own baby when she died. She cried as she remembered her baby, but found it very therapeutic to help her daughter carefully dress her. This repeating of a sad family event in the next generation had allowed her to grieve for her own loss.

Other relations

Depending on the extent of the family, there may be aunts, uncles and cousins who are very close to the dying child or to the parents. It may be helpful for hospital staff to be given a list of those whom the family has asked to visit.

Friends

Special friends may be very important at this time, sometimes more so than family. A child's godparents or childminder may have a close relationship with the child. The child may have a particular friend who wants to visit, or perhaps a friend who witnessed the accident. Friends who may not have seen the child for a while may need to be warned about changes in the child's appearance and abilities.

School

The child's school should be kept informed and appropriate messages given to classmates and friends. The teachers need accurate information to answer other parents' questions. This is particularly important if a child has meningitis, as other parents are always frightened that their child might 'catch' it.

CAUSES OF DEATH IN PAEDIATRIC INTENSIVE CARE UNITS

Some units offering intensive care for children specialise in particular types of surgery, such as cardiac, transplants (heart, heart/lungs, kidneys, liver) or neonatal surgery. These children are often critically ill, which means that a considerable number of children die whilst waiting for surgery or during the postoperative phase.

Some units operate a retrieval service so that a team can respond to a request for help from a child's local hospital. The team stabilises the child and transfers to the intensive care unit. This enables more children to benefit from specialist treatment and therefore to have a higher chance of recovery. If the child dies, the relatives are unfortunately further from their local support, but parents usually appreciate the efforts made to give the child the best care.

The biggest single cause of death in some general paediatric intensive care units is head injury. Head injuries may be also associated with multiple injuries in victims of road traffic accidents, or accidents involving bicycles or horses, or falls from windows, roofs or trees. Other main causes of death include: brain haemorrhage, cerebral hypoxia, meningitis, encephalitis, respiratory disorders (pneumonia, ex-premature babies with severe lung damage), sepsis, multi-organ failure, near drowning, poisoning and smoke inhalation.

Most of these causes are accidents or illnesses with a sudden onset; others might include a worsening of a diagnosed condition or an acute presentation of a previously undiagnosed condition, such as diabetic coma or leukaemia.

DEATH OF A CHILD IN ACCIDENT AND EMERGENCY DEPARTMENT

The A&E department is normally warned to expect a child being resuscitated by paramedic and ambulance staff. This gives time for paediatric medical and nursing staff to be prepared and for someone to be available to support the parents. Such situations include road traffic accidents, drowning, smoke inhalation, poisoning, severe burns and sudden infant death syndrome.

A critically ill or injured child may have a cardiac arrest whilst receiving emergency treatment in the department and this is extremely traumatic for parents to watch. Some parents prefer to wait outside, but many choose to see what is being done for their child. They need to know that everything possible was done and that the medical and nursing staff did not give up on their child. In this situation, it is essential to have an experienced member of staff to be with the parents, to explain what is happening and to prevent them from interfering with the procedures whilst distressed.

DEATH OF A CHILD ON A WARD

When children are critically ill with acute conditions, they will usually be transferred to an intensive care unit where they can be monitored and, if necessary, ventilated. Children who die on a children's ward in hospital are more likely to have been suffering from complications of a chronic condition such as cerebral palsy, hydrocephalus, heart, lung or liver disease, or one of the metabolic or degenerative disorders.

Death may be either sudden or expected. A child with a terminal illness or one who has no hope of recovery may be brought out of intensive care in order to have a more peaceful death, away from the high-tech equipment if that is no longer appropriate. A side room on the ward offers some privacy for the family but with the continuing support of the staff.

DEATH OF A CHILD AT HOME

Many children with life-threatening and terminal conditions are nursed at home with support from community staff. Special equipment may be loaned from the hospital or community nurses, such as suction machines and pumps for tube feeding or intravenous fluids and drugs. The family's general practitioner and hospital medical team will provide medical care, and community paediatric nurses offer guidance and support for the daily care. A baby-sitting service is available in some areas to enable a parent to have a few hours free to shop or spend time with other children.

The family may be able to visit a hospice for children if there is one near their home. Several hospices for children have opened during the past decade and offer respite care in order to give the parents a break. Parents may choose for their child to die there when the time comes, or the hospice outreach team may go out to support the family at home.

Some parents have an arrangement with the hospital to give them open access to the ward. This means that if the parents are concerned about the child, they can come straight to the ward without contacting their GP first. This may be very reassuring for them; parents might be managing to care for their child extremely well, but may feel less confident when the child's condition deteriorates. It is a huge responsibility to care for a dying child at home and at times carers can feel quite lonely. Support is needed for the family to be able to address the emotional as well as the practical issues.

PREPARING FOR THE DEATH OF A CHILD

One could argue that nothing will prepare parents and relatives adequately for the death of a child, but we should at least try. One way of getting at this question might be to differentiate between expected and sudden deaths, but then what do we mean by expected and how sudden is sudden? Even when a terminal illness makes death inevitable, we cannot be certain when exactly the patient will die, so the death may still come as a shock. An accidental death or brain haemorrhage would be sudden – one day the child is well, perhaps in school, the next day she is not. This could happen to any child of any age; it is always a shock and everyone feels vulnerable. The family is in shock, the relatives are often numb, and all are unable to believe that this is really happening to them.

Parents of a child with a life-threatening condition or who has been seriously ill for a while may be well prepared for the death. They may be relieved that the child will not be suffering any longer and know that they have done their best for the child. Parents sometimes try to rationalise the situation, for example, when a child has been brain damaged through a head injury or when the brain has been starved of oxygen. Some may not be able to imagine how they would cope with a child who is unable to behave normally, and make remarks like: 'He was always so active, he could not have coped with life in a wheelchair.' Others, perhaps being truthful about themselves, may admit they could not bear to see him survive and be severely handicapped.

Kübler-Ross (1969) has described grieving as a process of five stages or phases:

1. denial
2. anger
3. bargaining
4. depression
5. acceptance.

Although some professionals criticise this description of grieving, as individuals may not 'fit' the stages in the suggested order, the phases are certainly recognisable by an observer or helper and by those who are grieving. The feelings in these phases are relevant to anticipatory grieving in those alongside a dying person and to the dying person herself, as well as to people grieving after a death.

Denial

At first there may be a numbness, which gives a temporary protection to the parents against the harsh reality, but as this passes and they begin to understand the meaning of what the doctors have told them, they can feel quite isolated. The devastating news has somehow separated them from the normal and from their hopes. They may feel unable to talk to well-meaning friends and relatives, which adds to the feeling of isolation. The natural defence of denial often comes into play here and they may pretend it is not really happening to them. 'Wake me up and tell me it is only a nightmare' and 'I have to pinch myself to remind me that it is really happening' are two of the typical comments made by parents.

A feeling of uselessness is common in parents faced with this situation, as echoed by Spufford (1989), who also acknowledged a feeling of isolation. 'I know of the desire to be of use, in itself perhaps suspect, because it must be compensatory for the isolation which unusual experience brings'. At this point it is important to keep a steady contact with the parents. They may not be ready to talk yet and this must be respected, but leaving them alone may add to their sense of isolation.

Anger

This feeling is often very strong but hard to express or acknowledge (see also Ch. 3). It may become quite distressing and confusing for some parents. A parent writing after his child died said he could not explore the anger he still felt at his son's death, because he did not think it could be explained away, only experienced

(Stuart and Totterdell, 1990). He recognised that although he was angry because of the death, other inadequacies and frustrations had been exposed.

Parkes (1986) reminded us that grief is a process not a state, and that the expression of anger seems to change with the passage of time. His studies of widows showed that irritability and anger are a feature of the early phase of grief.

Bargaining

This is a short stage, perhaps a last attempt to postpone the inevitable. Most of the actual bargaining usually takes place in secret, trying to do a deal with God, perhaps with the chaplain or other minister, or privately. There may be a final plea with the doctors to try another drug or treatment. Counselling skills may be helpful to allow the person to reflect on and eventually accept the truth.

Depression (see also Ch. 6)

I prefer to use the word despair, in the context of anticipatory grieving, as it relates to the realisation of the loss of a future for the child and with the child. There is despair, too, among parents at the thought of how they will cope without the child.

Acceptance

I imagine that no one can ever totally accept the loss of their child, but they can perhaps accept the reality that it is going to happen or that it has happened already.

Totterdell (Stuart and Totterdell, 1990) speaks for many parents of sick and dying children when she pleads for doctors to manage the sickness but to let parents manage the quality of their own children's lives. To give some guidance through this difficult period, it may be helpful to use a few questions to enable the family to maintain some control over events and to make choices:

- *How?*
  - — *How* are we going to manage this situation? *How* will we cope?
  - — *How* long do we have? *How* long does the child have?
  - — *How* does the child feel?

- *What?*
  - *What* do the parents know and understand? *What* does the child understand?
  - *What* more can we do? *What* would the family like? *What* would the child like?
  - *What* has happened to change things?
  - *What* will happen now?
- *When?*
  - *When* do we talk again with the parents? *When* would be a suitable time?
  - *When* will they be ready?
  - *When* is the right time to stop treatment?
  - *When* is the child likely to die?
- *Where?*
  - *Where* is the most suitable place to nurse the child – at home, on a ward, at a hospice, in intensive care, in a side room?
  - *Where* are the siblings?
- *Who?*
  - *Who* would the child and parents like to have with them? *Who* should come? *Who* should not come?
  - *Who* would support them? It is important for the family to have the people they choose to be with them. It is a time to be natural and spontaneous, and not to feel they have to entertain visitors and continually explain the situation. Time with their child is limited and so the remaining time is precious and special.

CARE OF A DYING CHILD

The physical care of a dying child is desperately important and many parents like to feel that they are in control of this. However, some parents may not be in a state to make decisions or generate their own ideas, in which case it may be helpful for nurses or others to make suggestions.

The principal considerations are similar whether the child is being cared for at home or in hospital. Here are a few suggestions:

Dignity

The child and family should be afforded as much dignity as possible within the scope available. Superfluous equipment and unnecessary invasive monitoring can be seen as an intrusion into what should be a peaceful time. Parents need to understand what the equipment is for and agree to its removal. Not all parents feel the same way – most would prefer to have equipment taken away, but some choose to wait until the monitors alarm and the heart trace shows a straight line. They perhaps need that evidence of death or to witness the exact moment when the heart stopped.

At home, there would not be any monitoring equipment, although there may be a pump for drugs or feeding. Hopefully, the family would feel well supported in their decision to care for the child at home and in their choices for the child's comfort.

The family will usually appreciate attention to details in the care of the child. Even if they do not notice at the time, they may remember it later. Keeping the child clean is an obvious necessity, but washing hair, cutting nails, and wearing favourite clothes and hair bands are all important too.

Pain control

There is no reason for a child to suffer pain when a choice of many drugs and modes of administration will help. Parents ask repeatedly for reassurance that their child is not in any pain. They know the child better than anyone else and can recognise any change in expression or crying that might indicate discomfort. It is necessary for parents to feel that they have protected their child from unwanted intrusions when they have not been able to protect the child from dying.

Nutrition and fluids

Eating and drinking are essential features of life and many parents like to feel that a dying child is not being denied the comfort of favourite tastes if possible. A mother who is breast-feeding may decide to stop when her baby is dying as she does not want to be left with milk after the baby has died. Another mother may choose to continue, even if the milk is expressed and the baby fed by tube, because she wants to provide for the baby for as long as she possibly can. A dying child in an intensive care unit, even if unconscious, usually continues to have intravenous fluids until it is agreed to discontinue.

Family involvement

Time spent with a dying child is often considered very precious, especially when family members are able to share it together. If the child is aware of those around her, it is especially important to have them helping with care, reassuring and supporting. The parents, in particular, will be able to take some comfort in their loss, knowing that they did all they could for their child, for as long as they could. They did not 'give up' on their child.

Comfort

Comfort for the family while they care for the child helps during this difficult time, but comfort for the child is their main concern. Keeping the child warm, clean and dry are obvious requirements, but a careful choice of chairs, bed, mattress and bedclothes is also important. Many wards and intensive care units provide duvets, sheets and pillow cases in children's fabrics which are pleasing for the family and the child.

Familiar voices, music

Hearing seems to be the last of the senses to go, so it is always important to talk to an unconscious person if we cannot be sure that she can hear. The familiar sounds of parents' and siblings' voices is reassuring, helping the child to feel secure and not alone. Many parents like to play tapes of favourite music, songs or stories. It is not unusual to have recorded sounds of a school assembly, a class teacher reading, messages from friends or the family dog barking. When parents leave the bedside, they may play a tape through earphones so that the child does not feel alone.

Favourite soft toys

The feel of a cuddly soft toy is comforting for the child and the family. Siblings sometimes make sure that the favourite is on the bed; a good way of involving them is asking them to choose which toys to bring to the hospital. Most children have a special soft toy to take to bed, and it is often so much a part of the child's bedtime routine that parents insist it stays with the child to the grave. The nurses need to know of any important toys and to label them with the child's name.

Holding, stroking

Wherever a dying child is nursed, physical contact is important for the child, the parents, the family and the staff. If for some reason parents are not with their child at the time of death, most parents will want to know who was there and exactly what happened. It will be important to them to know that the child was not alone.

Parents may sit for hours just holding and stroking the child; it may be the only remaining thing they can do. Even if a child is in intensive care on a ventilator, it may be possible to lift the child onto the parents' laps to be wrapped in a soft blanket or quilt and held. The hospital bed can be lowered to allow a parent or sibling to lie on the bed beside the child.

EMOTIONAL CARE OF THE CHILD

Children who are dying as a result of an accident, following major surgery or from a serious illness with a sudden onset may not be aware that they are dying. Those who have lived with a life-threatening illness may have realised the possible outcome as they get older. This is particularly true of children with conditions such as cystic fibrosis or liver disease, where they may have known other children in hospital who have since died.

Children need to develop an understanding of their illness and Lansdown (1996) suggested that this develops in stages which follow the chronology of the illness. He identified five stages in children's developing understanding of their illness:

1. *I am ill.* This statement becomes real when they recognise the signs of illness such as missing school, visits to the doctor and hospital, taking medicines, not feeling as well as usual and perhaps not being able to do the activities they used to do.
2. *I have an illness that can kill people.* When they know the name of the illness, children can become aware that people can die from 'my illness'.
3. *I have an illness that can kill children.* An awareness develops that children can also die from 'my illness'. They may know of other children on the same ward, who attend the same outpatients clinic, special needs school or support group, who have become very ill and died.
4. *I am never going to get better.* They may have feelings of despair, that they have been ill, perhaps for a long time, and are not getting better.
5. *I am going to die.* Children may think that death is a logical conclusion to not getting better. Many children who are ill or in pain, even in a short acute illness with an excellent prognosis, ask if they are going to die.

Honesty

Most children today are unfamiliar with death in the family, and particularly the death of children, in the way that would have been common perhaps 100 years ago. However, as Lindsay (1995) reported, where children have experienced the death of a close relative or are themselves terminally ill, research points to an ability to understand death much earlier than mainstream accounts suggest.

Parents and other relatives may think it kinder to protect a child from the truth about the illness, but honesty is much easier for both the child and the family. If nobody mentions the subject, the child may not feel able to, and a barrier of pretence and denial will grow between the sick child and others whom the child needs for support. It is sad when a family are not able to share the final precious time together in an honest and trusting relationship which they can remember with love for the child. Children will generally find someone in whom they can confide about death and dying (Bluebond-Langner, 1978). They may ask the nurses deep questions that worry them if they feel their parents cannot bear to talk about it or will not give them truthful answers. The parents may have strong wishes that the child should not be told the prognosis. This could create a dilemma for the nurse trying to preserve a moral code of honesty (Heath, 1994).

An important factor to consider is the parents' own reaction to the truth about the child's condition (Peck, 1992). They may need more time to accept the fact that their child is dying before they are able to support the child in this knowledge. They may refuse to accept it and insist that treatment is continued, against medical opinion. There are many ethical approaches to making decisions concerning a child's right to be allowed to die (Ellis, 1992), but the courts have been involved in a few situations.

Those who work with dying children will remember some in particular who seem to be very aware of their impending death. Even very young children have asked for the light to be turned out, saying they are going to have a long sleep, or deliberately told parents that they loved them.

Some children have told of seeing a vision of happy children inviting them to play, or wanting to go into another room, or seeing themselves at the beginning of a tunnel with beautiful coloured lights at the end. Parents might be alarmed by such unusual stories and need to be reassured. The support and understanding of professionals are greatly valued at this time.

One 10-year-old was aware that the child in the opposite bed was dying even though no one had told him. He told his mother not to bring his cousin to visit as it was not right – did they not know there was a boy dying in there?

Children who are sufficiently aware of being seriously ill will probably be concerned about the future. They may feel increasingly isolated and thus in desperate need of a close loving relationship with the family and the staff, within which they feel safe to ask their questions. Hall (1997) reminded nurses that they need a sound knowledge base of related issues as well as practical confidence to be able to answer the dying child's questions.

CARE OF THE PARENTS

Health professionals who are caring for dying children and their families must be prepared for many and mixed emotions. Parents may experience feelings of numbness and disbelief, intense anger and guilt, blame and hurt, helplessness, hopelessness and desperation. There is not always time to prepare, if ever it is possible to prepare yourself for the death of your child, and carers may be the safest target for some of the anger and other feelings.

The importance of information

There may be conflict in parents' minds as to whether they really want to hear what the doctors tell them. Some parents have said how they 'hate that doctor' because he is the one who gave them bad news; what they meant was that they hated hearing what had to be said. But most parents stress the importance of being told the truth and not being given false hopes. Honesty and truth are essential for establishing trust and, at this time especially, they need to trust the professionals.

When giving information to the relatives, particularly bad news, it is usually helpful to start with what they already know and build on that. Ask when was the last time someone spoke to them, and what they said. Check if they understood what was said and how it affects the child's care now and in the time ahead. Remind them of earlier significant information; for example: 'You remember that yesterday we were getting worried about the swelling of Ben's brain. We had thought it might swell after the injury and we gave him all the support and treatment we could to try to prevent this getting worse. You know we have repeated the scan of his head this morning. I'm afraid it shows there has been no improvement; in fact his brain is more swollen. He is showing signs that his brain is not working, and whilst we are continuing to support him, I have to tell you that I do not think he will be able to survive.'

The response to this could be a desperate plea to continue and not to 'give up on him'. Mothers in particular may react by saying that they just want the child to survive at all costs, and, without thinking about what it might really mean, they may say they would cope with a brain-damaged child.

A question asked frequently is: 'What happens now?' Families need some idea of the time-scale in order to make their plans. They need to know that the staff work together as a good team and are all telling the same story. To check that the story is true, they may ask questions of everyone.

Whilst they will want to know what will happen, e.g. when and how the child will die, it is sometimes helpful to acknowledge that this could be a new and frightening experience for them. It is highly likely that they will not have seen anyone dead before and are afraid of how they will manage this.

In summary, information must be honest, accurate, appropriate, given at the night time, consistent and repeated if necessary.

Involvement in the child's care

Parents usually like to do as much for their child as they can. If they know that their time together is going to be limited, they put aside jobs that can wait, the priorities change and they want to stay nearby. Even in intensive care there are ways for parents to take part in the care – changing nappies, washing, eye care, mouth care and cleaning teeth are just a few. It is important to stress the parents' role in the team caring for the child, as they need to feel valued and understood.

Helpers should also be aware that for some parents, taking part in such activities may be more than they can bear. Washing a wasted arm or leg, cleaning a sore bottom or cleaning eyes that do not respond might be too distressing.

Regular food and drink

Parents may not consider their own needs for refreshment when the child is the priority, but terminal care is exhausting. They may not be able to manage large meals, but tempting snacks and fruit will help to keep up their energy. If they do not feel like eating much then at least they should be taken regular drinks. Relations and friends are often pleased to bring in food or to stay with the child while the parents go for a break to have something to eat.

Rest and sleep

Parents may think they can keep up a constant vigil with their child, but they do need periods of rest and sleep. In hospital, a time could be set aside when there are no disturbances, so that both parent and child can have a peaceful rest. Every encouragement should be given to parents to try to sleep.

Help with calls, visitors, press, police

It is often said that bad news travels faster than good news and sometimes a family can be inundated with telephone enquiries and visitors. Telling the same story to each caller becomes a chore, especially when the news is not good and there is no change to report. Ward staff may help families when they do not want to talk to everyone by filtering calls and taking messages if the parents would rather not come to the telephone. It is often helpful for a member of the family to relay information around the wider family instead of the parents having to talk to everyone. Occasionally, a friend or neighbour may be rather overpowering in a desire to help, and parents may ask for advice in keeping them away.

There is sometimes interest from the media, particularly the local press, when there has been an accident or incident involving a local child or family. Staff need to be aware of reporters making enquiries about the child or asking to speak to the parents. Some hospitals have a press office that deals with all press calls. When a family is shocked and anxious, they should not have to face intrusions from reporters or photographers.

The police may need to interview parents after a road traffic accident or other incident and every effort should be made to make this ordeal as simple as possible. When a seriously ill child has been brought to hospital by ambulance, the police may drive the parents to join their child as they may not be in a fit state of mind to drive a car safely or be able to get there quickly. The police may also be involved when a child appears to have suffered a non-accidental injury and physical abuse is suspected.

Help with other children and grandparents

Parents of a dying child often ask for help in talking to the siblings, perhaps because they do not know how to tell them what is happening, since it is too painful for them. They may also be afraid of their reactions and questions. Grandparents need help to understand the situation so that they can help to support the family. Again, the parents may not be the most suitable for this task, so staff should be available to talk with grandparents and other relatives.

Time to be alone, and alone with the child

Time alone is a precious space to think, to just 'be' rather than having to worry about what should be done next, or at least to think in peace about what to do next.

Time alone with a dying child is very special for most parents; it is an opportunity, possibly the last, to say whatever they want to say. In hospital, it is important to ask parents if they would like to be left on their own, as they may feel awkward about asking the nurses. They may, however, prefer to have the reassurance of constant attention from their nurse. Some parents are so involved with their child that they do not even notice who goes in and out.

Parents' own visitors

Parents need to have their own visitors. The focus of attention is on the child but parents need the support of their family and friends, adult conversation and news from the world outside the hospital or home.

Spiritual support

Spiritual issues are always aroused when someone close is dying. The parents of a dying child have the added responsibility of 'doing all they can' for the child. They may not have a faith them-selves, but sometimes want to make sure that this does not penalise the child. Parents have been heard to say they want the child christened or blessed by a minister of a church as a 'pass-port' to heaven. Most ministers would probably say it does not work like that and that God loves all children. Other parents may feel angry with God or will be unable to believe in a God who 'allows' children to die.

These feelings are very personal and are often kept inside, being too delicate to discuss with anyone else. Parents may feel comfortable talking to a hospital chaplain or their own minister of religion, who will certainly help many of them to sort out some of their thoughts. A counsellor will also allow parents freedom to explore, independent of a particular faith.

Families may reach a point of desperation where they are pre-pared to try anything with the remotest possibility of success, because that is all they have left. They may behave quite out of character and seek alternative medicine and faith healers.

A strong faith can be a tremendous support and guide in times of trouble and can also raise questions. Hospital chapels usually have comforting readings, poems and prayers for visitors to read, and offer a quiet place to sit and think or pray. Whatever a person's beliefs or philosophy of life, when they are facing the impending death of their child they need to be at peace with themselves and with those around them, especially the child.

CARE OF OTHER CHILDREN (see also Ch.11)

Other children involved with the dying child will usually be the siblings, step-brothers and -sisters and half-brothers and -sisters. There may also be school friends, neighbours or children who witnessed the accident.

What do they know and understand?

If children are not told the truth, they will probably make it up and their version is likely to be inaccurate. It is helpful to start with what children already know and to check that they understand it before telling them more. Their understanding, whether it is from what they have been told or whether it is made up, needs to be correct before they are confused by additional information which may not make sense (see Case Study 14.2).

CASE STUDY 14.2   *Children need accurate, age-appropriate information*

Maxine saw her friend knocked over by a car on their way home from school. She knew she was badly injured but some boys in her class were frightening her with horrifying tales that 'they' had chopped off her leg. Maxine telephoned the unit herself because she wanted to know if this was true.

What do they need to know?

Children need to be told the truth; at least they should not be told lies. Elsegood (1996) suggested these guidelines for telling children bad news:

- what has happened
- what is happening
- what is going to happen
- what this is likely to mean for them
- what is being done to help.

Who will tell them?

Children are usually helped most when given information by the adult to whom they feel closest and with whom they will have a continuing relationship based on a history of trust (Elsegood, 1996). Sometimes it is extremely hard for a parent to tell a child that a brother or sister is seriously ill and may not get better. They cannot bear to believe it themselves and may not be able to say the words. Children must have consistency in what they are told; everyone must tell the same story. This should be stressed to families.

Care should be taken in deciding when to give children bad news. The adults in the family may need time to sort out their own feelings first so that they are more prepared to help the children. It is advisable not to delay too long and run the risk of children hearing the information from other sources first, especially as this may not be correct. This will not help with the maintenance of trust within the family.

Children's concept of time should be considered when giving information. It would be distressing for the family if a young child went around telling everyone that a brother or sister was going to die, and then it did not happen for several weeks, or asked constantly if a sibling would die today.

School teachers have an important role supporting siblings and friends of a very sick and dying child. It is important for them to be kept informed so that they can help the children, again making sure the story is consistent.

Who is caring for them?

Parents need to know where their other children are staying and that they are happy. It is important for the adults caring for these children to be kept informed of the sick child's state of health so that the children's questions can be answered truthfully.

How can they be involved?

Children do not like to be left out, so talking with them in person or on the telephone helps them to stay in touch with what is happening. Involving them in decisions, and encouraging them to draw pictures, write stories and help with the sick child's care can give them a real sense of taking part.

Help them to visit

Children may need to have good explanations not only of what is happening, but also of what they should expect. Preparing them for what they will see and how the child will look is helpful. Visiting children may find visits difficult and they may only stay with the sick child for a few minutes at a time. This is understandable, as young children are easily bored and may prefer to play in the playroom. Children like to be made welcome in the hospital environment and little treats help to make them feel special too.

Give them time

Siblings of a sick child will want to spend time with their parents as well, to tell them their news, and may like to meet the nurses and others on the ward.

WITHDRAWAL OF TREATMENT

A time may come when active treatment is no longer appropriate and the care is aimed at giving the child a dignified and peaceful death back in the arms of the family. It is especially important that the family members understand completely what the medical and nursing staff tell them and that they are given sufficient time to discuss the situation. If they do not understand or agree with decisions taken at the time, their grieving afterwards can become more difficult.

In intensive care units, children are usually treated aggressively and given full support until such time as it is no longer considered right to continue.

If the prognosis is agreed to be hopeless and the child's condition deteriorates quickly despite full treatment, then most parents would agree to allow the child to die peacefully in their arms. But they have to be ready to share that decision with the doctors; they have to be certain that everything reasonably possible has been done for their child, otherwise they could live with the parental guilt of having failed their child. Paediatric intensive care units hold many promises but they can also hold unrealistic expectations and have the potential to dim moral vision (Purcell, 1997).

The best interests and welfare of the child are the primary considerations (Department of Health, 1989) and the ethical principles of beneficence, non-maleficence, autonomy and justice

(Beauchamp and Childress, 1994) provide fundamental guide-lines to ensure these interests are served. Nurses, midwives and health visitors are guided by their *Code of Professional Conduct* (UKCC, 1992) 'to act at all times to safeguard and promote the interests of individual patients'.

The Royal College of Paediatrics and Child Health (1997) has published guidelines on withholding or withdrawing life-saving treatment in children. These offer a framework for practice and should help parents as well as medical and nursing staff to feel comfortable with such decisions. Fundamental to this issue has to be that the child's best interests are served. In summary, these guidelines state:

There are five situations where the withholding or withdrawal of curative medical treatment might be considered:

1. The Brain Dead Child. In the older child where criteria of brainstem death are agreed by two practitioners in the usual way it may be technically feasible to provide basic cardiorespiratory support by means of ventilation and intensive care. It is agreed within the profession that treatment in such circumstances is futile and the withdrawal of current medical treatment is appropriate.
2. The Permanent Vegetative State. The child who develops a permanent vegetative state following insults, such as trauma or hypoxia, is reliant on others for all care and does not react or relate with the outside world. It may be appropriate both to withdraw current therapy and to withhold further curative treatment.
3. The 'No Chance' Situation. The child has such severe disease that life-sustaining treatment simply delays death without significant alleviation of suffering. Medical treatment in this situation may thus be deemed inappropriate.
4. The 'No Purpose' Situation. Although the patient may be able to survive with treatment, the degree of physical or mental impairment will be so great that it is unreasonable to expect them to bear it. The child in this situation will never be capable of taking part in decisions regarding treatment of its withdrawal.
5. The 'Unbearable' Situation. The child and/or family feel that in the face of progressive and irreversible illness further treatment is more than can be borne. They wish to have a particular treatment withdrawn or to refuse further treatment irrespective of the medical opinion on its potential benefit. Oncology patients who are offered further aggressive treatment might be included in this category.

In situations that do not fit with these five categories, or where there is dissent or uncertainty about the degree of future impairment, the child's life should always be safeguarded by *all* in the Health Care Team in the best possible way. Decisions must never be rushed and must always be made by the team with all the evidence available. The decision to withhold or withdraw curative therapy should always be followed by consideration of the child's palliative or terminal needs.

Many children who cannot be helped by continued treatment go home so that they may die with their family around them in the comfort of familiar surroundings. The Children Act (Department of Health, 1989) states that the child's welfare is paramount and particular regard is paid to the wishes and feelings of the child. Sometimes the child will make the decisions, which parents may find helpful (see Case Study 14.3).

CASE STUDY 14.3 *Sometimes children make the decisions*

Thomas had been sick for most of his 6 years. He had undergone major surgery the previous year and his condition had deteriorated once again. He looked thin and pale and was very tired. His parents were aware of his poor prognosis even with another operation. They asked Thomas what he would like to do next and he replied immediately: 'I just want to go home.' So that is what they did, and he died peacefully at home a few days later. His parents knew they had been right because it was what Thomas wanted; he had helped them to let him go peacefully, away from the hospital and all the invasive treatment, equipment, noise and routines.

CONCLUSION

The death of a child will remain a tragic, disturbing and possibly unacceptable event in a paediatric intensive care unit or children's ward. For some parents, the unit is a place of great hope, offering a chance of recovery with experienced care and advanced technical equipment. For others, it is where they come to realise that they are at the end of their hopes and their child is not going to get better. Sudden and accidental deaths of children are devastating for families, and they need time to make some sense and reality of what has happened. We should also have compassion for those families for whom the death may bring relief after months or years of anxiety and exhausting care, perhaps at home.

Susan Hill (1989) wrote a book about the long struggle for her premature daughter's life. As her baby was dying, she wrote:

Watching someone die of a grave, long illness, someone who is old but has had some good life, is hard, of course it is, but there is an element of acceptance in the onlookers as well, perhaps, in the dying person themselves.

But a child, a baby, whose time is not ripe, who has had no life yet to speak of, who has all hope, all potential, everything to come – it is impossible to accept, one's instinct is to hope against hope, to do battle, to fight for its survival, no matter what.

REFERENCES

Baum, J. D., Sister Francis Dominica, Woodward, R. (eds) (1990) *Listen, My Child Has a Lot of Living to Do – Caring for Children with Life-threatening Conditions.* Oxford: Oxford University Press.

Beauchamp, T. L. & Childress, J. F. (1994) *Principles of Biomedical Ethics,* 4th edn. Oxford: Oxford University Press.

Bluebond-Langner, M. (1978) *The Private Worlds of Dying Children.* Princeton, NJ: Princeton University Press.

Department of Health (1989) *The Children Act 1989.* London: HMSO.

Ellis, P. (1992) A child's right to die: who should decide? *British Journal of Nursing,* **1(8)**, 406–408.

Elsegood, J. (1996) Breaking bad news to children. In *Working with Children in Grief and Loss,* ed. Lindsay, B. & Elsegood, J. London: Baillière Tindall.

Goldman, A. (ed.) (1994) *Care of the Dying Child.* Oxford: Oxford University Press.

Hall, A. (1997) Talk to me, I'm dying. *Paediatric Nursing,* **9(8)**, 21.

Heath, S. (1994) Making decisions in clinical care. *Paediatric Nursing,* **6(9)**, 20–23.

Hill, L. (ed.) (1994) *Caring for Dying Children and their Families.* London: Chapman and Hall

Hill, S. (1989) *Family.* London: Michael Joseph.

Judd, D. (1995) *Give Sorrow Words – Working with a Dying Child,* 2nd edn. London: Whurr Publishers.

Kübler-Ross, E. (1969) *On Death and Dying.* London: Tavistock/Routledge.

Kushner, H. S. (1981) *When Bad Things Happen to Good People.* London: Pan Books.

Lansdown, R. (1996) *Children in Hospital – a Guide for Family and Carers.* Oxford: Oxford University Press.

Lindsay, B. (1995) Like skeletons or ghosts: developing a concept of death and dying. *Child Health,* **2(4)**, 142–146.

Parkes, C. M (1986) *Bereavement – Studies of Grief in Adult Life.* London: Penguin Books.

Peck, H. (1992) Please don't tell him the truth. *Paediatric Nursing,* **4(2)**, 12–14.

Purcell, C. (1997) Withdrawing treatment from a critically ill child. *Intensive and Critical Care Nursing,* **13**, 103–107.

Royal College of Paediatrics and Child Health (1997) *Withholding or Withdrawing Life Saving Treatment in Children – a Framework for Practice.* London: Royal College of Paediatrics and Child Health.

Spufford, M. (1989) *Celebration.* London: Fount Paperbacks.

Stewart, A. & Dent, A. (1994) *At a Loss – Bereavement Care when a Baby Dies.* London: Baillière Tindall.

Stuart, A. & Totterdell, A. (1990) *Five and a Half Times Three, the Short Life and Death of Joe Buffalo Stuart.* London: Hamish Hamilton.

Wilkinson, T. (1991) *The Death of a Child – a Book for Families.* London: Julia MacRae Books.

United Kingdom Central Council for Nursing, Midwifery and Health Visiting (UKCC) (1992) *Code of Professional Conduct,* 3rd edn. London: UKCC.

FURTHER READING

Brenkley, W. (1991) Understanding bereavement. *Paediatric Nursing,* **3(1)**, 18–21.

CRUSE-Bereavement Care (1993) *Supporting Bereaved Children and Families.* London: CRUSE.

Department of Health (1989) *The Children Act 1989: an Introductory Guide for the NHS.* London: Department of Health.

Herbert, M. (1996) *Supporting Bereaved and Dying Children and their Parents.* Leicester: BPS books.

Hindmarsh, C. (1993) *On the Death of a Child.* Oxford: Radcliffe Medical Press.

Jewitt, C. (1982) *Helping Children Cope with Separation and Loss*. London: Batsford.

Lansdown, R. & Benjamin, G. (1985) The development of the concept of death in children aged 5–9 years. *Child: Care, Health and Development*, **11**, 13–20.

McHaffie, H. & Fowlie, P. (1996) *Life, Death and Decisions, Doctors and Nurses Reflect on Neonatal Practice*. Hale: Hochland and Hochland.

Neuberger, J. (1987) *Caring for Dying People of Different Faiths*. London: Austin Cornish.

Stannard, D. (1995) You can show you also care. *Nursing Standard*, **9(37)**, 54–55.

Walker, J. (1990) Care in bereavement. *Paediatric Nursing*, **2(8)**, 17–19.

Wells, R. (1988) *Helping Children Cope with Grief – Facing a Death in the Family*. London: Sheldon Press.

Widdrington, C. (1992) Preparing for loss. *Nursing Times*, **88(49)**, 26–28.

Supporting bereaved families

INTRODUCTION

A bereavement is usually understood to be an enforced loss of some kind. In the context of this chapter it refers to the loss of a child and all that was part of life with that child. The family members feel robbed; they have been deprived of a life, and of the hopes for the future that went with that life, and are left desolate. When a child dies, parents experience the loss of a uniquely significant relationship (Rubin, 1993). Parents may suffer the death of a child of any age – even when that child is an adult. At the other end of the age scale, we have stillbirth and neonatal death, both of which are shocking experiences (Jones and Jones, 1990), and sudden loss can also result from miscarriage, termination or abnormality. If carers and health professionals can develop an understanding of bereavement and be prepared for the range of emotions and mixed reactions that may erupt, they will be better able to help.

I suggest there are four periods of bereavement during which support is needed:

1. Before the death, if possible
2. At the time of the death
3. Immediately after the death
4. A longer time after the death.

DURING THE PERIOD BEFORE THE DEATH

Grieving begins with the diagnosis, when the 'bad' news or information is received. For families with a sick child this may be:

- Congenital abnormality – grieving is for the normal baby that was expected and for the lost hopes and aspirations.
- Genetic disorder – parents grieve for the normal baby they could not have because of the inherited condition they have

215

passed on. The feelings of guilt and failure can be powerful and may become an enormous burden.

- Accident or injury – there will have been little or no time to prepare and parents may have feelings of guilt, blame and anger as well as shock at what has happened.
- Onset of severe illness – babies and children may become seriously ill very quickly and the shock of a life-threatening illness gives rise to parental feelings of failure and guilt.

Chapter 14 explores the care of the family in more detail, but Box 15.1 provides a summary of the main considerations.

Box 15.1   Main considerations when caring for the family of a dying child

- *Information* – honest, appropriate and carefully timed checking parents' understanding at all stages
- *Time* – for the child and family to ask questions, to talk, express fears and allow feelings to come out
- *Siblings* – give honest information; involve them
- *Emotional support* – from those who will listen and share; support from professionals
- *Social support* – from family and friends
- *Spiritual support* – from a minister or hospital chaplain; importance of rites such as baptism, blessing and anointing; time alone
- *Physical support* – food, drink, rest; caring and anxiety are exhausting

---

AT THE TIME OF DEATH

It is helpful if the wishes of the family are discussed with the medical and nursing team before the child dies, so that necessary preparations can be made and the family supported. Religious or cultural issues may be significant at this stage or just after the death. Sensitive observations and enquiries will help the staff to judge the extent of their involvement at this time. Most parents would like their child to die in their arms; even quite large children can be placed on parents' laps or alternatively a parent could lie on the bed and cradle the child. The family might prefer to be on their own with the child or they may like to have nurses around them.

In an intensive care unit or accident and emergency department, a child's death may occur after dramatic resuscitation attempts, where the child is surrounded by many people and much equipment. If the parents witness the resuscitation, there should always be a professional there to support them throughout the procedure and explain what is being done to the child. When a death is sudden, it is usually helpful to have seen how hard people tried to 'save' the child. Parents who have witnessed resuscitation attempts often say they did not like being there but that it was important to see that everything possible had been done.

Cot death, or sudden infant death syndrome, is devastating for parents and distressing for all involved: an apparently normal baby is found not breathing, most commonly early in the morning. The family will be shocked and disbelieving, especially the mother, or whoever was caring for the baby, who may be hysterical and taking all the blame and responsibility for what has happened. The baby will normally be brought by ambulance to the accident and emergency department of the local hospital, where the staff will be ready to receive him into the resuscitation room. The apparently overwhelming grief and distress may cause the ambulance personnel to bring the baby to hospital alone (Wright, 1991). Both parents should be encouraged to come to the hospital as soon as possible.

When resuscitation attempts have failed and the medical team withdraws, most parents like time to sit and hold their baby. Specimens of blood, urine, stool, spinal fluid, and swabs for culture from nose, throat and skin will be taken at this time. Parents may question these procedures and it may be helpful to explain the need to try to find out the cause of the baby's death. The doctor will take a detailed recent history from the parent or whoever is at the hospital, although this could be very distressing. The family should be warned that a police officer will interview them, but reassured that this is normal policy and does not mean that the parents are under any suspicion.

A doctor must confirm that the child is dead and note the time in the patient's notes. The exact time that the heart stopped may be important for the parents to remember.

IMMEDIATELY AFTER A CHILD HAS DIED

This is a special time for parents and attention to the detail of their wishes is important. Good care at this stage will help them in the difficult time ahead. A hospital chaplain (Morris, 1988) has suggested his own 'Five Ts of bereavement first aid':

1. *Touch* – I am real, you are real, this experience is real and not a dream. He/she is still and unresponsive, beginning to get cool. You cannot let go of what you have not been able to grasp.
2. *Talking* – 'Tell me what has happened' – articulating the unimaginable helps to make it real.

3. *Tears* – 'Auto-pharmacology' – swallowed tears give the stomach something other than its own lining on which to work. They trigger the production of endorphins, which help to induce calm and relaxation.
4. *Tea* – or other non-alcoholic drink replaces lost body fluid consequent upon adrenalin surge, and eases the hangover headache of dehydration. An everyday activity of making and drinking tea helps re-orientate the shocked and numb.
5. *Time* – has run out for the dying/dead/bereaved. Time spent in companionable silence lets them know that they are still special. Proper support *at the time* of bereavement can save months of individual and family anguish later.

After a child has died, the family members may be feeling confused, exhausted, relieved, desperate, frightened, hysterical and angry, among many other emotions. It is therefore helpful if professionals are prepared for these mixed reactions and are aware of their own feelings at the time.

Parents may become anxious about what they have to do next, but there is no rush; they should take all the time they need. The nurses' calm and continuing attention to the family can encourage them to make the most of this special time. Some parents like to have a while on their own, whereas others do not like to be left without a nurse, so it is helpful to check regularly which they would prefer. They may not know what they can do or ask for, so they may appreciate some suggestions and guidance. Parents usually appreciate encouragement to hold their child until they are ready to wash and dress them.

Washing and dressing the child

Parents may prefer to leave the nurses do this, as they do not all choose to help. However, the physical contact of being able to wash their child for the last time is a healing and therapeutic experience (Stewart and Dent, 1994). There might be some particular task that a parent wants to perform – perhaps washing the child's hair, bathing the baby, putting on a nappy for the last time, using a favourite soap or dressing the child in a special out-fit. It is often very important for parents to feel they can still make choices and care for their child. It is during this period, after their child has died, that they will slowly begin to appreciate fully what has happened. They will be aware of the cooling and stillness and change in colour; many parents are able to say that the child is not there any more. If the nurses and other staff are able to feel comfortable about maintaining a naturally gentle and continuing contact with the family, then the family will be more able to feel comfortable and calm.

Keepsakes

Parents may not be able to think for themselves and make decisions, so it is helpful to ask if they would like any photographs taken, or a lock of hair to keep. They may like to cut this themselves (a useful hint is to tie a lock of hair tightly with tape or a band of sticky tape, quite close to the head, and cut between the tie and the head, thus keeping the strands together).

Photographs provide a way of preserving a visual memory of a moment and professionals may be surprised by some of the photographs parents take. Many families like to have photographs of their dead child, to keep private or to show to other family members who were not present. They may take close-up pictures of parts of the body, such as hands and feet, and take photographs of the child with each sibling, parent or grandparent. It may be important to remember anyone who is not present such as a parent who is not living with the child.

All the family can share in making prints of hands and feet; the brothers and sisters usually like to help. An inkpad or coloured paints can be used to make prints on plain paper or cards. The strands of hair could be stuck inside the card with sticky tape.

Other items that parents and siblings have asked to keep include wrist name-bands, labels from above the hospital bed, and drawings, cards and letters from siblings and school friends. Staff may be surprised at what is important for parents to keep. Some time after a child has died following a road traffic accident, a parent may ask what happened to a shirt or pair of shoes that the child was wearing that day. The staff may have decided, because the shirt was bloodstained and had been cut off on arrival in the accident department, to dispose of it. But for the parent, this was the last garment the child wore; it might even have been the child's favourite shirt. It may even be important to them precisely because it does have the child's blood on it; in a strange way it is proof that the child was badly injured, making this dreadful nightmare real.

A family may be too distraught to decide if they would like any keepsakes, or it may be that owing to other circumstances members of the close family are not present. Staff could take photographs, hair and handprints, keeping them safe in an envelope in the notes until a suitable time. Parents may not feel able to take photographs home at this time, so again they can be kept until they are ready to be taken.

Time to say goodbye

This opportunity to say goodbye should be given to brothers and sisters as well, whenever possible, so that they can see for themselves what they are leaving. If they are not told the truth or given the opportunity to see for themselves, their fantasies may be worse than the truth. A 14-year-old sister once remarked, after seeing her dead brother, that she felt better now she had seen him – she had wanted to see 'what they had done to him'. She had not imagined that he would look so peaceful. Some family members may be keen to move on to talk about funeral plans, but that can wait if this period of time is precious.

The time immediately after a child has died is often extremely hard for the staff caring for the family, whether the death was expected or sudden. Sometimes it is more than the family can bear and, in their distress, the parents may want to flee. The staff need to be sufficiently skilled and confident to be able to support and encourage them to take their time to say goodbye, to begin to accept that their child is dead. At the time, letting the parents go may seem the easiest and kindest approach to protect the family from the pain, but in the days, weeks and months ahead the parents may have considerable difficulty in accepting that their child is not coming home. They may also have regrets about not staying, and feel guilty that they let down the child at the end.

Organ donation (see Ch. 9)

When parents have consented to their child being an organ donor, it is usually particularly significant for them to see the child after the retrieval operation. Otherwise their last memory is of the child being pink and warm, on a ventilator, with the chest going up and down as though breathing. It is helpful for them to see the child peaceful, pale and still. If kidneys only are being donated, the child may be taken to theatre immediately after a doctor has confirmed asystole.

Death at home

Most children who die at home have been suffering from a long-term illness and families may be well prepared for the death. It may be a shock and a relief at the same time and family members benefit from experienced help and guidance through what they need to do. It is usually possible for the child's body to remain in the home until the parents are ready for the undertakers to remove it to their chapel of rest. If the family wishes to keep the body at home until the funeral, the undertakers will give the best advice on this. They are available at any time of the day or night, which is important for parents to know, in case they change their minds and prefer the body to be taken out of the house.

Postmortem examinations

Parents must give their consent for a postmortem unless a coroner has requested one in order to establish the cause of death. The consultant in charge of the child's care may not have a definite diagnosis or cause of death and may ask the parents' permission for a post-mortem to give further information. If the parents do not give permission and the doctor cannot give a cause of death then the coroner could be consulted and may request a post-mortem. In some situations, a doctor may ask the parents if a postmortem could be performed in order to find out more about the child's condition, either for the parents' own information or to contribute to research into the condition.

Some parents do not like the idea of any further intrusion and make comments such as 'He's been through enough'; however, many will agree, hoping that any information obtained might help other children. It may be helpful, if appropriate, to explain to parents that although they may not want to ask questions now, in a few days, weeks or months they may want to know some details that can only be answered by a postmortem examination. By then it will not be possible to give these answers. An alternative solution is to perform a limited examination, in which only stipulated parts are examined; for example, one could examine the heart of a baby with a congenital heart condition or the abdomen of a child with liver disease to establish the extent of the involvement of other organs.

Parents should be reassured that they will be able to see the child's body afterwards, and that it will be stitched as after any surgical procedure.

'What happens now?'

Most parents will not have experienced a death in the family and will be anxious about what they have to do, so they will look to the staff for guidance. Some sort of booklet or information sheet that can be taken home is helpful; it is not sufficient simply to give information verbally when people are tired and shocked. The information that is needed is presented in Box 15.2.

Box 15.2   Information to be included in a leaflet for parents whose child has died

- Some acknowledgement of their loss, such as: 'We are very sorry that your child has died and would like to offer you help in any way we can. At this distressing time it may be difficult to think about what you need to do, so we hope this information will be useful.'
- An explanation of the medical certificate of the cause of death – this gives the cause(s) of death and the medical diagnosis and will be written by one of the doctors. If there is to be a postmortem examination to establish the cause of death, or if the coroner is to be notified, then the certificate will not be issued straight away.
- An explanation that the coroner will be notified of all accidental, sudden or unusual deaths, and may contact the parents.
- Reassurance that the child's body will be cared for – 'We will look after your child until your funeral director has made the necessary arrangements. If you would like to come and see him/her in the Chapel of Rest at the hospital, this can be arranged. Please telephone the ward or patient affairs office to discuss this. It may be possible for you to take your child home and we can discuss this if you wish.'
- An explanation of how to register the death – a death must be registered in the town where the death occurred, within five working days, usually by a parent or relative. If the coroner has been informed, then the family will be advised by the coroner's office. Parents will need to know the address and telephone number of the local registrar of births, deaths and marriages and when to ring for an appointment. A map showing the location of the office will be helpful for those not familiar with the area. If a baby's birth has not been registered, this must be done at the same time.
- Contact telephone numbers at the hospital – ward, chaplain, counsellor, social worker, patient affairs office.
- Telephone numbers of national and local support organisations such as CRUSE Bereavement Care, Compassionate Friends, SANDS (Stillbirth and Neonatal Death Society) and Child Death Helpline.
- Some suggested books they might find helpful.

Other useful information to give in an envelope could include leaflets from support organisations, some information on the feelings and emotions to expect in grieving, and children's responses to a death in the family.

Remember also to check the following with the parents *before they leave:*

- Do they have transport home, preferably with someone else driving? If not, ask if they are fit to drive. Offer them somewhere to sleep if they are tired and have a long journey.
- Make sure their home or contact telephone number is recorded.
- Make sure they take all their belongings with them.
- Ask them if they would like the hospital staff to contact anyone for them, such as a relative, a neighbour or the child's school.

- Check that they have the medical certificate of the cause of death or instructions about collecting it the next day or if they know that the coroner will be contacting them (if appropriate).
- Check that they have been given any information leaflets available.
- Do they understand how to make arrangements to see the child again?
- They should be reassured that they can telephone at any time for help of any sort or simply to talk to someone.

Guidelines for professionals

It is usually helpful if some guidelines on managing the death of a child are prepared and kept where they may be found easily and used for reference by staff not familiar with the procedures. When a death occurs during the night or at a weekend, it is not that easy to ask someone who knows what to do. Staff new to the ward or hospital may not be familiar with local policies and procedures. Distressed parents value the support of professionals who are aware of what they might need to be told, as they may be feeling too upset and tired to ask questions or express their wishes. They will expect guidance from those around.

The guidelines should include important points for nurses caring for a dying child, the medical staff and the family. The following information should be included:

- The doctor confirms the death and writes it in the patient's notes.
- The medical certificate of the cause of death (usually incorrectly called the death certificate) can be written by a doctor on the ward unless the diagnosis is unclear and a postmortem examination is required or the coroner is to be informed.
- The location of the book of certificates and an explanation of how to use it. Write the main part of the certificate, tear it out and put it in an envelope addressed to the registrar of births, deaths and marriages. Seal the envelope and attach the 'notice to informant' slip which was part of the page in the book. Fill in the stub in the book. Give the parents a copy of a map or instructions to find the registrar's office. For babies dying within the first 28 days of life, the book of certificates for neonatal deaths must be used.
- The doctors writing the certificates should print their names and contact bleep or telephone numbers in case there is a problem. Some medical conditions are not acceptable by the

registrar as a cause of death and a list of these would be helpful with the book. It is very distressing if parents go to register the child's death and are told that the doctor or the coroner will have to be informed before this formality can be completed. Give contact numbers for advice on wording.

- If a certificate is not being issued, the doctor must explain to the parents either (1) that the coroner is being informed and they will be advised by the coroner's office when a certificate will be issued; or (2) that a certificate will be issued, perhaps by a doctor who knows the child better, or after medical discussion as to the correct diagnosis or cause of death. The parents would be advised when to collect the certificate.
- The coroner must be informed of any sudden, accidental, suspicious or unexplained deaths, or if a patient died during or soon after an anaesthetic or operation. It should be remembered that some patients (such as those with head injuries) may die some time after an accident, but the death is as a result of an accident and must be referred to the coroner. Permission for removal of organs for transplantation is usually given by the coroner. Record the names and telephone numbers of the coroner and coroner's officer. The police may also need to be informed since the death could affect their charge (e.g. causing death by dangerous driving).
- Where to find necessary forms such as consent for postmortem examinations, necropsy requests, consent for organ donation.
- Hospital policy for labelling bodies.
- Policy for transferring bodies to the mortuary.
- Policy for dealing with patient's notes, X-rays etc.
- People to inform, including:
  — consultant if not involved at the time
  — any other medical staff or professional involved in the child's care
  — general practitioner
  — health visitor or midwife
  — referring ward or accident and emergency department
  — referring hospital
  — coroner?
  — social worker?
  — police?
  — patient affairs office.

This is a long list of important points to remember, but knowing where to find helpful information at a difficult time is supportive for staff. It helps them to feel in control of the situation and of themselves, which in turn helps the families who need supportive guidance. Bereaved families need information to be given in a clear and confident manner, and it should be written down so they can take it home to read it again.

Other parents and children on the ward or unit

It is important to consider the other children and their families who are on the ward at the time of a death, particularly those who knew the child. The parents may have talked about their children to each other and so some will be well aware of the situation. Most parents are upset when a child dies on the ward while their child is also a patient. They feel vulnerable, especially if their child is also very sick or has a similar condition; they are faced with the truth that children do indeed die, despite all the medical and nursing care, technology and equipment.

In an intensive care unit, for children or babies, there is often a strong bond between parents. They are all sharing the same feelings and concerns and they can be deeply affected by a death; some even express guilt that their child has survived and another has not. Confidentiality must be respected, but alongside this must surely be a responsibility for the care of other families. Parents might ask a nurse: 'What happened to Ben? Did he go home?' A truthful reply is needed. In an intensive care unit, where the children may be nursed in a close environment, it may be appropriate to tell the parents simply and quietly what has happened. It is not easy to tell parents of other sick children that a child has died, but they usually appreciate being told the truth rather than being left wondering and imagining. It also gives them the choice of whether to remain in the unit while the family of the child who died are crying and while there may be extra visitors. They may ask if they should go outside while the family members are distressed or when the body is removed; the staff could check this with the grieving family. Needless to say, different people have different views on this. I have seen a mother become quite angry that another mother remained sitting by her own child's bed, saying: 'You would think she would have gone out at a time like this.' However, most parents say that the others need to be with their children, and more often than not, because they are so involved in what is happening to them, they are oblivious to everyone else.

Some children may need to be told about the death of another patient, particularly if they knew the child well. Many children with chronic life-threatening conditions such as cystic fibrosis or liver disease will know other children with the same illness and it is hard for them to learn of the death of someone with whom they shared a special bond. Older children might ask questions about the cause of death: 'Was his chest bad?' or 'Did she die after the operation?' These could be significant to their own situation, and perhaps to the way they come to terms with the possibility of death. Questions like this show that they are being realistic about their condition, treatment and prognosis.

Some unusual circumstances

There are times when parents are not present at their child's death, adding to the distress and anxiety. If a child is critically injured whilst a passenger in a vehicle involved in a road traffic accident, there is a possibility that a parent or sibling will also be injured. The victims might be brought to hospital in separate ambulances, or even to different hospitals. The parents may be unconscious or needing emergency surgery themselves and it may not be possible for them to be told the devastating information about their child's condition or death. They could be desperate to find out what happened to the child or children and they need honest answers; it is not fair to avoid their questions (see Case Study 15.1).

CASE STUDY 15.1   *Giving injured parents the opportunity to say goodbye*

Jenny and Alex and one of their boys were in their car when it was in a head-on collision with another vehicle. The boy died in the car at the scene of the accident and both parents were badly injured and taken to hospital where they were admitted for surgery. Jenny and Alex were in beds next to each other in a side room, to offer them some privacy on a busy surgical ward. The following day, they desperately wanted to see their son, to see for themselves that he was dead, in order to believe what they had been told. It was not possible for them to be taken to see their son's body in the chapel of rest, as they were on large beds with traction equipment, so the child was taken to them.

A nurse and the chaplain prepared the child in the mortuary, put him in a bed with bedclothes from the children's ward and took him in the service lift to the parents' ward. The bed was placed between the parents, with the beds lowered to the same height. The child was lifted gently to be close to each parent in turn, but held by the professionals as the parents were too weak. They stroked him, held his hand and talked to him, saying how sorry they were about the accident.

This time was very special for the parents and they told family and friends later how important it had been. They remembered details of what the child had been dressed in, saying that it was what he would have chosen, and also the children's prints on the duvet. This operation had not been easy for the professionals; good teamwork and trust between the mortuary staff, coroner's officer, ward staff and the chaplain and nurse was essential.

Planning the funeral

Many parents of dying children will have had thoughts or fantasies about the funeral before the child has died, even if it has been hard to talk about it (Goldman, 1994). This anticipatory grieving and planning can be helpful, as a way of coping with the uncertainty of waiting for the death and of accepting the inevitable outcome. Nurses and others around the family at this time may find this hard to understand, especially when the parents' discussion is followed by expressions of guilt for thinking about a funeral while the child is still alive. Reassurance that this is perfectly natural may allow them to express their thoughts; it is, after all, only trying to continue caring and doing their best for their child.

Included in the planning for the funeral may be thoughts about having the child's body at home for some or all of the time until the funeral. For some parents this is an invaluable period (Stuart and Totterdell, 1990), perhaps because they cannot bear to leave the child with someone else, even after death. It is important to advise parents to contact the funeral directors, who can help them with arrangements for keeping a body at home, such as room temperature, and who are available day and night.

Some parents may have definite ideas about the funeral, while others need to ask for help. They should be given the time and attention to make the occasion appropriate for them. Some funeral directors take special care to make a child's funeral different, offering coloured coffins with pictures, paying attention to the needs of brothers and sisters and involving family members in the service. Parents may choose to carry the coffin into church or to the grave themselves – the final act they can do for their child.

A LONGER TIME AFTER THE DEATH

Continuing support for bereaved families needs to extend beyond the death and the funeral for as long as it is needed. Some families seem to need help for many months and years, whereas others prefer to grieve in private and do not seek any help. Everyone is different and there are no right and wrong ways to manage grief.

I believe that bereavement care should be in the community – where the family and friends live and where their future lies. However, we must recognise that the hospital has had a special role for the families and they may not be ready to 'let go' of the team that cared for their child and supported them through the death. Following a lengthy illness in their child, parents can be bereaved by the loss of hospital personnel and activities, as well as other parents (Brewis, 1995).

Remembering the funeral

A funeral is an important 'rite of passage' which allows an opportunity for sharing sadness, expressions of grief, offering thanks for the life now ended and saying farewell individually and collectively. Some health professionals may like to attend a child's funeral, to say their own goodbyes and to show support for the family. A card to say they are thinking of the family is usually appreciated if no one from the health care team is going to be present.

A follow-up appointment

Some bereaved parents like to return to the hospital very shortly after the child's death, but for others a space of a month or two usually gives time for questions to surface. If the child was nursed at home, then the general practitioner and the community nurses will visit the family and offer available support. In our unit, the consultant and I send a joint letter inviting bereaved parents to meet us both for an appointment, giving the date, time and place. This letter should be worded sensitively, explaining the purpose of the meeting and offering to meet at a later date if this is too soon.

Hospital staff must not underestimate how hard it might be for parents to return to the place where their child died. I usually start a session by acknowledging this. In reply, parents often reveal that they have not been sleeping properly of late, as they were dreading coming in and even having nightmares and flash-backs. They may have powerful memories of previous visits to the hospital – the clinic appointment when the fateful diagnosis was given, the emergency rush to hospital trying to follow the ambu-lance, the sound of the siren and parking in a hurry. They deserve some recognition for meeting this challenge and coming in.

Parents usually feel more at ease if the meeting place is not a room with bad memories, such as the doctor's office where bad news was given to them. It is also helpful if interruptions from telephones and bleeps can be prevented. Offering some structure to the session at the beginning may help parents to use the time: 'We have about an hour with you now, which we hope will give you a chance to ask questions about David's illness. We have brought along his medical notes to remind us of the details. We would like to hear about how you are feeling now and if we can help in any way.' Make sure to offer coffee or tea as well.

Some parents bring a long written list of questions to be answered, and apologise for asking 'silly questions'. For many, the last day of their child's life is just a muddle of memories, and they often remember very few facts. Some parents still need to ask the fundamental question: 'Why did my child die?' The medical and nursing notes are helpful in putting pieces into the jigsaw and giving a more complete picture. It does seem to be a significant help in the process of grieving to be able to ask questions – as one mother put it 'to sort things out in your mind, to know that everything was done for her, that I have not failed as her mother'. The feeling of responsibility and guilt after a child dies may be strong, and parents need reassurance from those who were professionally and not emotionally involved. There may be late test results or postmortem reports to discuss, giving more valuable information for completing the 'picture'.

One of the reasons for this meeting is to see how the family has been coping since the death, and naturally they might be rather tearful during this return visit (so do not forget to have tissues handy). Parents often talk freely, knowing that those in the room with them are aware of what they have gone through because they were there too. For many it can be a relief to be able to talk about the death, instead of trying to protect friends and family from the details. It may be possible to suggest particular help from local or national bereavement support organisations or help for children from psychologists, family therapy or school. The family doctor will be able to help and advise on sleeping, eating and health problems that often present in bereavement.

Parents might ask about other children or members of staff in the unit at the time when they were there; the memories of friendship from other parents and appreciation for the care given by the staff can be strong. Before the parents leave, it is worth asking if they would like to visit the place where their child was nursed and died. Some may respond immediately and definitely that they could not bear to go there again, but for many this is important.

It is sensible to check beforehand that it is a suitable time to take them in – not while the staff are too busy to notice them, or while there are procedures or doctors' rounds in progress. A thoughtful tip is to note which patient is in 'their child's' bed-space – whether the current occupant is of the same sex, similar size or with similar equipment around – and to warn the family about this. This is important to them, and they may say, for example, they were relieved to see a baby where a 12-year-old had been, or a girl where a boy was. Some parents comment that they 'had to see his bed just to be certain that he was not still there'. For some, it is necessary to see that the ward or unit continues to be there for other children.

The offer to return may not be taken up; many parents do not reply, but it does seem important to leave open the possibility of a visit at a later date.

Continued links with the ward

Many bereaved parents, grandparents, other relations and friends want to give something back to the ward, unit or community service in gratitude for the care given, but also in memory of the child. Tremendous efforts may be put into fundraising, and while this is valuable to the recipients it must not be forgotten just how important it might be for the fundraisers. This is something they can actually do in a practical sense and it can relieve the feeling of helplessness in the face of a child's death. It is a tribute, not only to the child who has died, but also to the family, who feel comforted and supported by the attention. A plaque with the child's name and a message such as 'Given by the family and friends of ...' serves as a physical reminder of the child. Some parents of children being nursed in intensive care have said that they feel slightly uncomfortable seeing plaques 'in memory' of a child on equipment being used for their own child, but in general it is considered a positive thing, for which people are grateful.

Bereaved families sometimes visit the ward on a particular day, such as the child's birthday, the day they died or perhaps at Christmas if they had spent a Christmas in hospital.

Individual support

Grieving is a very personal matter and however strong a partnership between parents, each is an individual with individual needs and ways of dealing with grief. There will be times when they seem poles apart and times when they understand each other without needing to speak. When two people are grieving deeply, it can be difficult for them to help each other, perhaps because they are struggling to help themselves and have no energy left for each other (Wilkinson, 1991).

'Grief work' has been defined by one bereavement counsellor as the three 'e's – 'to *endure*, consciously *experience*, and *express*'

(Kander, 1990). Individual support and counselling may help someone to explore thoughts and feelings at any stage in the grief process. It might be shortly after a death or many years later (see Case Study 15.2).

CASE STUDY 15.2   *Unresolved grief*

Marjorie was being treated for depression by her general practitioner who was exploring her past medical history. He made enquiries about bereavement counselling at the hospital when it was revealed that Marjorie's son had died 14 years ago, aged 3. She accepted readily the invitation to a session with the consultant paediatrician and nurse counsellor at the hospital, during a telephone call to discuss what she would like to do. Marjorie was very keen to come for herself and understood her husband's decision not to come.

The child's hospital notes had been found and brought to the meeting; Marjorie was surprised they still existed and it made her cry to see his name written down after so long. She had many questions about the child's illness and treatment and why he died, and asked if treatment today would be different. The doctor went through the records very carefully, as there were gaps in her memory that she needed to fill.

Marjorie felt reassured when it was suggested that she had only relatively recently allowed herself to grieve for her child who had died many years earlier; she was not becoming 'a psychiatric case' as she feared. She was able to agree that she had been kept so busy bringing up her three other children that her own grieving had been 'put on hold'. It was only now that these children were older and were asking questions about their brother that Marjorie's unresolved grief became apparent. She had needed to return to the hospital, to meet this paediatrician who was able to refer to the child's medical notes and answer fundamental questions about his illness and treatment, and to see where he died.

Marjorie was most grateful for the visit, saying how much she had learned and that she felt much better. Her general practitioner wrote to the hospital to express his thanks, feeling that this mother could now move on to live a happier life. From a health professional's perspective, some valuable observations may be made:
- The GP realised that unresolved grief could be a possible cause of depression.
- He enquired about available help.
- The paediatric department at the hospital understood the importance of offering a visit; bereavement follow-up visits are offered routinely.
- There were professionals available with the skills to help.
- A session of 1.5 hours was offered to the mother, with suggestions as to how this might be used. This eased her anxiety about what the session would be like – who would be there, where they would meet, how long she could have and what she could talk about.
- There was good teamwork between the GP and the hospital.
- The mother was made to feel valued, that grieving was a normal reaction to the loss of her child, which she had 'postponed' while she was fully occupied with her other children.
- A single visit of 90 minutes with two skilled professionals helped this lady more than frequent visits to her doctor and antidepressants. The GP's 'diagnosis' had been right and he had found good resources to support him.

Sometimes, a couple or a whole family can be helped during a single session, but sometimes they need more than one visit. A family group is a good forum for everyone to say how they feel, with a counsellor as a safe facilitator. Grandparents may also ask for help; they have their own needs, perhaps feeling helpless in trying to support their children and grandchildren.

Groups for bereaved parents

Some bereaved parents like to meet others who have lost a child, often for the simple reason that they cannot believe that anyone else will be able to understand the feelings they have. A bereaved parents' group can be supportive because it offers a safe place to share the experiences, thoughts and feelings of people who do understand. One bereaved father commented that through losing his child he now belonged to the most exclusive club, but with the highest entrance fee. Groups are not for everyone – many parents prefer to stay amongst family and friends and not try to meet new people at this time. But many families are not supportive and many friends do not know how to help, so not only have the bereaved parents lost their child, but they may have lost relationships and friendships at a time when they need them most.

I have found that it is helpful to hold a group for recently bereaved parents, whose child died within about the last 6 months, to offer some support during the early months when feelings are raw and the family members are struggling to manage their lives. Parents may still be distraught, with feelings of fear and guilt – 'man's greatest enemies' (Kübler-Ross, 1983). Kübler-Ross reminded bereaved parents that 'all the guilt in the world is not going to help a soul, least of all it is not going to help your child who died. Guilt will make you sick emotionally and, if you don't let go of it, physically'. I must stress the importance of having experienced facilitators for these groups as I cannot overstate the power of the emotions which are present and the sensitivity required to be able to hold the group together and to hear what is being said.

People usually feel more comfortable in smaller groups, perhaps up to 10 people, but larger groups can be divided. I have been with some groups of just four or six people who have found it really hard going with so few, while others have been highly successful.

A pattern that I have followed for several years is to hold a series of four or five evening meetings for parents who have lost a child within the previous 6 or 7 months, but not normally within the past month. These meetings are held weekly, in a venue with comfortable seating, facilities for making tea and coffee, easy car parking, and in a part of the hospital which is 'neutral' ground for parents who may find it hard to return to the hospital. A letter inviting parents to attend is sent from the three professionals who arrange the group, giving all the information and a tear-off slip for their reply. Some parents appreciate being offered a telephone number to talk with a group facilitator before they decide to attend.

The moods and dynamics of the groups vary according to the members, but the general opinion of parents and the helpers is that it is worthwhile. When parents are asked to evaluate their experience of a group, they may reflect on the pain of telling their story and listening to others' stories. They often say they learnt a lot about themselves and about grieving, and that it has been helpful to discover that they are not alone and that their reactions to the loss are natural and normal. Friendships can develop, the group may like to continue meeting in each other's homes and they are invited to a long-standing bereaved parents' group. It seems helpful for newly bereaved parents to have the opportunity to explore the raw feelings in a small group of parents who are at a similar stage in their grieving, before joining a group of parents who are 'further on'.

It is interesting to observe changes in individuals during the sequence of meetings; the sharing of their experiences and feelings with others is valuable. One father said that he had imagined that all children who died were killed in car accidents until he heard the stories from other parents. Parents whose child died after a long illness such as cancer can appreciate their last special weeks during the terminal phase when they hear from others whose child died suddenly in an accident or from a sudden illness such as a brain haemorrhage or meningitis. Those who lost their child suddenly may then feel spared of a long drawn-out death. Hearing other parents talk about their experiences in the group certainly helps them to feel they are not alone in their grief, and it is touching to witness how caring they can be in their thoughts for others. The group facilitators should be careful to warn parents at the first meeting that they do not have to take on the burden of other people's grief, as they have enough of their own.

From experience of running our own groups, I would suggest the following be considered:

- The letter of invitation is important.
- Groups should be small.
- Provide tea and coffee as the parents arrive.

- Have suitable books and poems available to read.
- Give opportunities for parents to show photographs of their children.
- Offer some structure to the course so they know what to expect.
- Give some simple theory of grieving, as it helps them to understand some of their feelings and to know that it is normal behaviour.
- Ask if there are any particular issues they would like to discuss, or information they would like. Time can be allocated for these.
- Address issues around coping with family occasions without their child – Christmas, birthdays, holidays.
- Give contact telephone numbers for local support organisations and helplines.
- Give a list of suggested books, articles and poems to read, perhaps written by other bereaved parents.
- Offer individual support during the course of meetings and afterwards.
- Acknowledge that both parents may not be able, or choose, to attend and one parent is welcome.

Remember also that other sources of support are available; some of these are given in Box 15.3.

Box 15.3 Other sources of support

- Support organisations
  — *CRUSE Bereavement Care* – a national organisation offering support, advice and counselling to anyone who is bereaved at anytime. Local branches
  — *Compassionate Friends* – an international organisation run by bereaved parents for bereaved parents. Offers a lending library service and sibling support. Local branches
  — *Child Death helpline* – operated by bereaved parents
  — *SANDS (Sudden and Neonatal Death Society)*
  — *Relate*, or other couples counselling – everyone grieves in their own way and couples are often torn apart by misunderstanding when they need each other
  — *BODY* (British Organ Donor Society) – for those involved with organ donation
  — *other support or self help groups specific for the illness or condition of the child.*
- General practitioner – counselling may be available through the practice
- Social Services
- Local churches
- Counselling organisations
- School – nurse, teachers for siblings
- Genetic counselling
- Family consultation clinic – for family therapy or individual work with children

Siblings

Bereaved brothers and sisters also need help and support through this difficult and confusing time (see Ch. 11).

Other children

Other children and young people who were part of the child's life must also be remembered – these are often the 'forgotten mourners' (Pennells and Smith, 1995). If the child was part of any group, such as a playgroup, school, sports team, ballet class, Brownies or Scouts, then all the others in the group will have their own needs. A particular loss may be publicly shared or suffered privately by an individual child (Capewell, 1996). They need to be told the truth about what happened and be given time to talk about the child who died and share their feelings with those who understand. School teachers have an important role in supporting children through what is often their first experience of the death of someone they knew.

Some problems with grieving

Mourning can sometimes 'go wrong', perhaps because the bereaved person is denying or postponing his grief so that his mourning cannot even begin. Grief can also be prolonged to the extent that a person cannot let go of the deceased, and is unable to move on in the mourning process. There may be a history of earlier losses, separations or trauma, leaving open wounds, or the person may be afraid, or may refuse, to let go. Feelings of anger, resentment, bitterness, guilt or revenge may be too strong to allow any progress to be made. A study by Summer et al.(1991) concluded that parents who lose a child in the intensive care unit constitute a high-risk group for psychiatric disturbance. Skilled interventions are usually helpful, through counselling, psychotherapy, assessment by psychiatrist and, possibly, use of antidepressant drugs.

CONCLUSION

I remember a phrase that a mother used when we were talking soon after her child had died. She said: 'We shall need all the help we can; we have not been this way before.' I thought about these words afterwards and realised the significance of 'this way' and 'before'. She sounded like someone about to set out on a perilous journey, down a route she did not know, and she was right to acknowledge the need for help.

The journey through bereavement follows a long uncertain route; there is no map to show the way, the steep difficult climbs, the slippery slopes or the obstacles in the road. There are not many signposts to show how far you have come or how much further there is to go, and you do not even know when, or indeed if, you will ever reach the destination. To continue the metaphor, a journey usually feels safer and less arduous when you have a companion. Sometimes the luggage feels a very heavy burden and it is easier when someone helps you to carry the load.

The special kind of help which that mother sought requires the helpers to be informed and prepared. This means having an understanding of what grief is about and, fortunately, there has been much written and studied on the subject (Kübler-Ross, 1969; Parkes, 1986; Worden, 1991). Kübler-Ross (1969) described five stages in the process of grieving, which are applicable both to those who have someone close to them who is dying and to those mourning after a death:

1. denial
2. anger
3. bargaining
4. depression
5. acceptance.

Tschudin (1997) reviewed many previous studies, and suggested that stages, frameworks and models have their place, giving helpers the possibility to work more effectively by not having to start at the beginning each time. Much has been written on 'stages' of grief and most researchers would agree that these are to be taken only as general flexible guidelines (Stroebe, Hansson and Stroebe, 1993). These authors also remind us of the stage theories of Bowlby (e.g. 1981) and Horowitz (1986). Bowlby's is a theory of attachment and Horowitz's is one of stress, these concepts being the most central and critical for the prediction of outcome or adjustment.

Grief does seem to be a process, and as with any process, the subject will pass through changes on the way. Worden (1991) described the tasks for the bereaved before they can expect to adapt to life without the deceased:

• to accept the reality of the loss
• to work through the pain of grief
• to adjust to an environment in which the deceased is missing
• to emotionally relocate the deceased and move on with life.

Parents who suffer the death of their child will have had their lives changed for ever. Nothing could be more hurtful than to be told 'you will get over it'; they do not want the child written out of existence (Dominica, 1987). They may, in time, be able to build a new relationship with this child and move on with their own lives. The words of a bereaved mother in one of our groups describe this:

> *'He may be frozen in time, but he is locked warm in my heart for ever, and no one can harm him or take him away now.'*

REFERENCES

Bowlby, J. (1981) *Attachment and Loss, Vol. 3 Loss: Sadness and Depression.* Harmondsworth: Penguin.

Brewis, E. (1995) Issues in bereavement: there are no rules. *Paediatric Nursing,* **7(9),** 19–22

Capewell, E. (1996) Planning an organisational response. In *Working with Children in Grief and Loss,* ed. Lindsay, B. & Elsegood, J. London: Baillière Tindall.

Dominica, Mother Francis (1987) Reflections on death in childhood. *British Medical Journal,* **294,** 108–110.

Goldman, A. (ed.) (1994) *Care of the Dying Child.* Oxford: Oxford University Press.

Horowitz, M. (1986) *Stress Response Syndromes.* Northvale, NJ: Aronson.

Jones, A. & Jones, K. (1990) Support for parents after a child's death. *Nursing Standard,* **4(46),** 32–34.

Kander, J. (1990) *So will I Comfort You.* Cape Town: Lux Verbi.

Kübler-Ross, E. (1969) *On Death and Dying.* London: Tavistock/Routledge.

Kübler-Ross, E. (1983) *On Children and Death.* New York: Collier Books, Macmillan.

Morris, I., Rev. (1988) *First Aid in Bereavement – Five Ts.* Unpublished lecture notes, Addenbrooke's Hospital, Cambridge.

Parkes, C.M. (1986) *Bereavement: Studies of Grief in Adult Life.* Harmondsworth: Penguin.

Pennells, M. & Smith, S. (1995) *The Forgotten Mourners – Guidelines for Working with Bereaved Children.* London: Jessica Kingsley.

Rubin, S. (1993) The death of a child is forever: the life course impact of child loss. In *Handbook of Bereavement: Theory, Research and Intervention,* ed. Stroebe, M., Stroebe, W. & Hansson, R. Cambridge: Cambridge University Press.

Stewart, A. and Dent, A. (1994) *At a Loss – Bereavement Care When a Baby Dies.* London: Baillière Tindall.

Stroebe, M.S., Hansson, R.O. & Stroebe, W. (1993) Themes in bereavement research. In: *Handbook of Bereavement, Theory Research and Intervention,* ed. Stroebe, M.S., Stroebe, W. & Hansson, R.O. Cambridge: Cambridge University Press.

Stuart, A. & Totterdell, A. (1990) *Five and a half times three – the Short Life and Death of Joe Buffalo Stuart.* London: Hamish Hamilton.

Sumner, M., Dinwiddie, D., Matthew, D. J. & Skuse, D. H. (1991) Loss on a paediatric intensive care unit: parental reactions. *Care of the Critically Ill,* **7(2),** 64–66.

Tschudin, V. (1997) *Counselling for Loss and Bereavement.* London: Baillière Tindall.

Wilkinson, T. (1991) *The Death of a Child – a Book for Families.* London: Julia MacRae Books.

Worden, J.W. (1991) *Grief Counselling and Grief Therapy,* 2nd edn. London: Routledge.

Wright, B. (1991) *Sudden Death.* London: Churchill Livingstone.

FURTHER READING

Bending, M. (1993) *Caring for Bereaved Children*. London: CRUSE-Bereavement Care.

Elliot, P. (1997) *Coping with Loss, for Parents. (How to Help your Child series)*. London: Picadilly Press.

Davey, N. (1995) Paediatric bereavement care. *Paediatric Nursing*, **7(9)**, 24.

Dent, A., Condon, L., Blair, P. & Fleming, P. (1996) A study of bereavement care after a sudden and unexpected death. *Archives of Disease in Childhood*, **74**, 522–526.

Dyregrov, A. (1991) *Grief in Children – a Handbook for Adults*. London: Jessica Kingsley.

Herbert, M. (1996) *Supporting Bereaved and Dying Children and their Parents*. London: Pandora/SANDS.

Hill, L. (ed.) (1994) *Caring for Dying Children and their Families*. London: Chapman and Hall.

Jewett, C. (1982) *Helping Children Cope with Separation and Loss*. London: Batsford.

Kohner, N. & Henley, A. (1991) *When a Baby Dies*. London: Pandora/SANDS.

Kushner, H. (1982) *When Bad Things Happen to Good People*. London: Pan Books.

Lindsay, B & Elsegood, J. (eds) (1996) *Working with Children in Grief and Loss*. London: Baillière Tindall.

Murren, E. (ed.) (1995) *Our Children, Coming to Terms with the Loss of a Child*. London: Hodder and Stoughton.

Raphael, B. (1984) *Anatomy of Bereavement – a Handbook for the Caring Professions*. London: Unwin Hyman.

Rosen, H. (1986) *Unspoken Grief – Coping with Childhood Sibling Loss*. Lexington: Lexington Books.

Rothman, J.C. (1997) *The Bereaved Parents' Survival Guide*. New York: Continuum.

Sarnoff Schiff, H. (1977) *The Bereaved Parent*. London: Souvenir Press (E&A).

Soutter, J. & Bond, S. (1994) A strategy for caring for families in bereavement. *Nursing Times*, **90(30)**, 37–39.

Wells, R. (1988) *Helping Children Cope with Grief – Facing a Death in the Family*. London: Sheldon Press.

Wright, B. (1986) *Caring in Crisis – a Handbook of Intervention Skills for Nurses*. Edinburgh: Churchill Livingstone.

16

Supporting the staff

INTRODUCTION

Health professionals involved in the care of sick children may be subjected to many varied problems and stresses. There are occasions when they can share in the happiness of a family whose child is restored to good health, especially after a serious illness or injury, and they can take some reward for their hard work. But they also share the sadness and disappointments of families. The death of a child may be a loss for them too. Winnicott (1986) claimed that:

It is doctors and nurses who experience reduplicated and repetitive mourning; one of the hazards of our professional life is that we may become hardened, because the repeated losses of patients makes us wary against getting fond of the newly ill. This is especially true of nurses who care for sick babies...

Nurses working with children face many stressors, especially when they are sick, injured, abused or dying, and it is not possible to hide from them. These nurses need to be well supported. Experienced nurses may have found ways of relieving their stress, including someone who they can talk to and with whom they can share their feelings. Less experienced nurses may be overwhelmed by events and the emotions they create, and may feel they should be coping alone. This invariably leads to a sense of inadequacy and of having failed the patient or family.

Some children with chronic or life-threatening conditions need help from many different professionals, so there must be a multidisciplinary approach to caring for sick children and their families. This may be true whether a child is in hospital, visits as an outpatient, attends a school for children with special needs, or is cared for at home. Effective teamwork helps to reduce interpersonal barriers and encourages peer support; it is important for the family to feel that everyone is working as a team – and that they are part of that team too. Everyone in the team needs support in this often extremely stressful work.

BEING VULNERABLE

Many adults involved with children will be rather vulnerable at times. The sick child could be the same age as their own child, the situation could be similar to their family, and they may have had a recent bereavement, miscarriage or divorce. Working with sick and dying children makes us question not only our own vulnerability but also our own mortality. If these young children can get so sick, have accidents and perhaps die, then so can we.

Many experienced nurses would agree with Lewis (1998), who argued that:

As individuals and as nurses it is important to recognise that in any situation our personal feelings will be present. An ability to cope with loss and change at work is dependent on our individual ability to identify, explore and come to terms with our own feelings so that they may be put aside in order that we can really listen to what others are saying.

Jung (1933) wrote that:

The relation between physician and patient remains personal within the framework of the impersonal, professional treatment ... you can exert no influence if you are not susceptible to influence. It is futile for the doctor to shield himself from the influence of the patient and to surround himself with a smoke-screen of fatherly and professional authority.

It does therefore seem sensible for doctors to allow themselves to acknowledge their own feelings and to recognise what is happening in the relationship. They are, as Jung suggested, involved personally, so will have their own emotions too. Wright (1986) also wrote about this personal involvement of staff in their patients' lives:

The crises experienced by our patients are not limited to them. The crises become a part of our work, and for a time, part of us. It is hoped that we will emerge from these experiences as agents of care who are able to facilitate change and direction in crisis.

LIVING UP TO A PROFESSIONAL IMAGE

Many professionals in health care survive the risk of being vulnerable by hiding behind a kind of mask or image of what is expected of them. For example, nurses wear uniforms and doctors have stethoscopes around their necks, and they all behave in a certain way in front of their patients. This 'professional manner' is not a bad thing; indeed, it is often reassuring for the patient and family because it is what they expect.

Jourard (1971) warned of the risks of patients being exposed:

...not to human beings who have expertise, but to 'experts' who are dehumanised and dehumanising. To spend time in the company of those who will not relate at a human level cannot be health engendering, either for the patient or the professional.

Jourard went on to observe that it seems to be difficult for professional healers to accept the fact that they cannot know any other person until they have taken steps to find out who and how they are. Psychotherapists would think of this as the other person's 'self' and 'how they are experiencing the world'. Put more simply, we should allow ourselves to have an empathic understanding of our patients and their families and to run the risks of entering into their 'world' briefly.

STRESS

The *Concise Oxford Dictionary* (1990) gives many definitions of this frequently used word, and the following four are relevant in the context of this book:

- demand on physical or mental energy
- distress caused by this – suffering from stress
- emphasis – the stress was on the need for success
- stressful – causing stress, mentally tiring.

Caring for sick children and their families can be very demanding of physical and mental energy. It can also be distressing to witness the suffering and strain of others, especially when the outcome cannot be described as successful. There is little published material on the stress that nurses experience as a result of working with sick children and their families (Jolley, 1995).

Not all stress should be considered to be 'bad', as a certain amount is normal and can help to motivate, such as when taking an examination or making decisions. Burnard (1991) offered the following definition of stress for health professionals: 'psychological, physiological and/or spiritual discomfort that is experienced when environmental stimuli are too demanding or exceed a person's coping strategies'. He added that we are constantly responding to stimuli, and that stress can be caused by stimulus overload, lack of stimulus or inappropriate stimuli.

Fortunately, we all have different ways of experiencing our lives, which means that we do not have the same reactions to, or coping strategies for, certain circumstances.

The problems of stress amongst carers demand attention, otherwise there are likely to be higher rates of staff sickness and absenteeism, low morale, dissatisfaction with the work and increased wastage of skilled people. This adds more difficulties when staffing levels are too low with poor skill mix and inadequate support from experienced staff and senior management. As Burnard (1991) wrote:

The business of working in the health professions means that we are constantly being exposed to stress. That stress can sometimes be enriching and motivating ... positive or negative; when it is negative, it is a problem. Working with other people who are troubled is indeed stressful. For too long it has been assumed that health professionals should 'get on with it', and put up with any stress that is involved with caring for others.

In hospitals particularly, there are many distressing sights, foul smells, unpleasant procedures to perform, complicated equipment to handle and anxious relatives to talk to, which all contribute to increasing personal stress levels. There are many routine and mundane jobs to be performed, such as monitoring and charting, which can be a welcome task or a source of irritation when there is other work to do. There may be high levels of anxiety, due to the constant fear of making an error of judgement or in technique in an area where mistakes could have fatal results.

Menzies Lyth (1959) wrote: 'By the nature of her profession the nurse is at considerable risk of being flooded by intense and unmanageable anxiety.' She described the way in which the hospital situation protects the nurse from this anxiety, for example: 'through splitting the nurse's duties between several patients, moving nurses from ward to ward, depersonalising the patients, through an expectation of professional and emotional detachment, and through performing ritualised tasks.'

This 'social defence system' helps the individual to avoid anxiety, uncertainty and guilt. As it matches the psychic defence system of the nurse, both continue to support each other through a continuous process of projection and introjection, but it does not allow growth or maturation in the nurse. This, Menzies Lyth suggests, may contribute to the high wastage of nurses.

A study by Harding (1996) looked at the main causes of stress for trained nurses caring for children with cancer and leukaemia, how they managed those stresses and how they could be helped

> **Box 16.1**   Main causes of stress for trained nurses caring for children with cancer and leukaemia, in order of decreasing importance (Harding, 1996)
>
> - Diagnosis
> - Parents
> - Shortage of nursing staff
> - Death/terminally ill children
> - Relapse
> - Seeing the worst cases/not successes
> - Nursing staff relationships
> - Relating to own children
> - Doctors
> - Causing the child pain
> - General running of the ward.

to manage better. The main stresses he found are listed in Box 16.1, in order of importance.

Staff working with sick children in different areas will have different significant causes of stress:

- *Staff in accident and emergency departments* may witness the horror of a badly injured child being rushed in with distraught parents and then have to pass the child on to the operating theatres, intensive care unit or ward. They are the family's vital first contact with the hospital and later may appreciate the opportunity to enquire about the child or visit her and talk with the parents. Resuscitation attempts that do not have successful outcomes are distressing for all present.

- *Community nurses* could feel isolated and lacking in support from other health professionals unless there are regular team meetings and opportunities to share information and concerns. They may feel sad and deprived when a patient they help care for at home has to go into hospital.

- *Ward nurses* may have similar feelings when a child goes home for terminal care and, although they know that this is the family's wish, they may regret that they cannot continue caring for the child during the remainder of her life. Children's wards often appear rather chaotic, with toys and activities around, babies crying, anxious parents, and for some, a sense of being rather public. New nurses may feel frustrated and unable to get everything organised. Staff on some wards may feel 'the poor relation' when they make comparisons with other areas that have higher staffing levels, more equipment and better facilities; the resulting frustration and dissatisfaction add to their stress. Many nurses who are not used to paediatric wards will find the parents stressful, having to involve them in all aspects of the child's care and feeling that the parents are watching them with their child.

• *Paediatric intensive care units (PICUs)* are stressful places for all staff who work there. Good teamwork is essential, with adequate support available for the individual needs of everyone. The ward clerk needs to have sufficient information about the children before she answers the telephone to distressed relatives. The cleaner needs to know why the floor must not be cleaned right now, when a child is dying, before it is thought that the person in charge is just being awkward. Things change quickly and staff must respond quickly, so trust in each other and sharing of tasks are important.

• PICU staff often feel that the very nature of their work is stressful, along with the uncertainty of what each day may bring. The workload can swing from being extremely busy, with the unit full of children each requiring very complicated care from more than one nurse, to having none or only one patient. When the staff are working under pressure, there are not the opportunities to leave the unit for breaks, as they work around the needs of the patient, and it may be difficult to keep up the charts and written work. Fears of making errors in drug calculations, fluid balance or interpretation of medical instructions add to the stress. Supporting the family of a critically ill child is often emotionally exhausting for staff who are also responsible for the clinical judgements and bedside care.

• The separate role of a counsellor with PICU experience has been shown to be beneficial to patients, families and staff (Cook, 1993). Other nurses have concluded that there is sufficient evidence from the available literature and their own findings to employ a counsellor/psychologist on units to deal with many problems, not only for parents, but also for staff (Colville, 1998; Curran, Brighton & Murphy, 1997; Lewis, 1998; Wesson, 1997). A counsellor provides a safe and non-threatening environment in which emotions may be more easily expressed. Some people suggest that the counsellor should also be a nurse who is familiar with the area of work, but some prefer an 'outsider'. Staff members are relieved to know that they do not have to carry all the family's emotional burdens and that they also have someone to listen to them, in confidence and without judgement.

Stress factors at work

The working environment is frequently a cause of stress, with such problems as having too many tasks to do at the same time, the demands of anxious parents, not enough space, too hot or too cold, unreliable equipment, delays in getting things mended, poor cleaning and housekeeping, noises from telephones, alarms and vacuum cleaners, and concerns about staffing levels and skill mix. Security has become an issue of concern for parents and staff. Many wards for children and babies have installed closed-circuit television monitoring and/or security entry systems to prevent unauthorised entry. Working with people is also often stressful, especially with parents who could be labelled 'difficult', staff who do not communicate with others in the team, senior staff who do not seem to be listening when help is needed, and characters who are aggressive or rude. It is not easy to tolerate anger from someone who appears to be aiming it at you, or who is verbally abusive when you are trying to do your best.

MANAGING STRESS

Supporting the staff through stressful times at work is not a luxury, but should be an integral part of caring for the child and family. Good members of staff are precious and should be valued and seen to be valued.

Encouraging self-awareness

It is helpful for individuals to learn about themselves, to listen to themselves and to think about what elements of their work they find hard to face and may even try to avoid. The same is true for different kinds of characters amongst people we work with or meet; thinking about the personalities and acknowledging to ourselves little things that annoy us or that we do not like usually make us more tolerant.

Before we can learn to manage stress better, we have to identify what makes us feel stressed, i.e. what causes a stress reaction. Many organisations run stress management workshops and there are books to help. There is much that individuals can do to help themselves, either on their own or in a group.

Exercise

Take a sheet of paper and divide it into two columns. In the left-hand column, make a list of everything you find stressful at work, then anything at home that is stressful and then what sorts of people (or any particular people) make you stressed.

In the right-hand column, write down what you might do to help manage each of the problems. Make aims that are realistic and achievable.

Ways of managing stress

If stress accumulates and becomes unmanageable, there is the risk of 'burn-out' or being unable to go on with work. This may present as an emotional breakdown or as physical symptoms such as gastro-intestinal disorders, malaise and apathy, aches and pains, nausea, raised blood pressure, loss or gaining of weight, headaches, sleep disorders, chest pains or palpitations. Colleagues may notice changes in mood, irritability, oversensitivity, crying, poor concentration, loss of interest in work, tiredness and not wanting to come to work.

Health professionals working with sick children and families must accept that their work is stressful and that there are times when, for various reasons, they are more vulnerable. In order to survive, they need to take care of themselves.

Boundaries

I think one of the first considerations must be the balance between work time and personal time – where the boundaries are drawn and how firmly they are fixed. Of course, there are occasions when our personal boundaries need to be pushed out a bit further; it is part of working in this field in which events cannot always be predicted. If staff offer to work extra shifts to cover for sickness then they must be sure they are not too tired to work extra time and claim the time back or be paid for it.

Time off is meant to be 'off', which should mean doing something different. Holidays are always important; the planning and anticipation of breaks have great value. We need something to look forward to, to keep us going!

The National Association for Staff Support (1992) has produced a *Charter for Staff Support*, for staff at all levels in the health care and social services. It acknowledges that the personal effects of occupational stress on the individual can be devastating in terms of physical and mental health and suggests that much of this stress can be prevented by:

- recognising that stress exists
- acknowledging the need for support
- educating staff in prevention and management of stress
- providing adequate support services
- creating a caring culture in the workplace
- promoting good staff support practices throughout the system.

The charter suggests existing services that could be used for staff support, such as:

- occupational health services
- counselling services
- chaplaincy departments
- in-service training courses
- 'time out' arrangements
- peer support groups
- good communication
- educational departments
- good management
- a good environment.

Education

Teaching the skills that are necessary to perform well in the role and which help in managing personal difficulties has more than one purpose – to enable the person to do a good job and to boost self-confidence and coping abilities. Many hospitals and community health trusts offer in-house study days and workshops for such subjects as: basic counselling skills, crisis counselling, communication skills, self-awareness and stress management.

Continuing in-service teaching should be available to further professional development and increase knowledge. Good information and resources for learning encourage interest in the subjects, and in return the professional grows in confidence as knowledge increases and the patient receives a much better quality of care. It is interesting to observe how much more acceptable support seems to be when it is labelled as training or education, with the emphasis on helping staff to do a good job better.

Interpersonal skills

The way we relate to one another and react to each other's actions and words have the potential for stress. Burnard (1990), addressing a consultation day for Project 2000 interpersonal skills in nurse training, discussed what these skills might be, how nurses viewed their own interpersonal skills, why they were needed and how they could be taught. He suggested the following list of necessary interpersonal skills, which I suggest are essential for most people in the 'caring professions':

- basic counselling skills – listening, attending, skilful use of questions, reflection, empathy

- assertiveness skills – for our patients and for us to be heard
- group facilitation skills
- skills in coping with other people's emotions
- telephone skills
- skills in caring for yourself
- skills in supervising and caring for others.

Burnard added that we also need to be able to make sure that the process of becoming more involved in other people's lives does not make for burn-out and emotional exhaustion.

TEAMWORK

Most people who work with sick children and their families are part of a team or even several teams. It may be a ward team, a community team, a multidisciplinary team or perhaps a nursing team, depending on the situation at the time. On a children's ward, there are many different personnel, including nurses of various grades, medical staff of various grades – paediatricians, surgeons, nursery nurses, hospital play specialists, physiotherapists, dieticians – social workers, school teachers and assistants, ward clerks, cleaners, chaplain, community staff and voluntary helpers. It really is helpful for building strong teamwork if everyone knows who everybody is and what each person's role involves. Understanding the strengths, skills and weaknesses of members of the team enables individuals to be valued and allows for the best use of the skills available.

Social events such as meals out, parties, picnics, games and visits to the theatre and concerts can help team members to get to know each other away from the working environment. Those who live alone or who are new to the area may welcome the opportunity to go out in a group. However, some people will prefer not to meet colleagues socially and to keep time free for their family.

INDIVIDUAL SUPPORT

As a counsellor and counselling supervisor, I realise the value of counselling supervision. The British Association for Counselling (BAC) states in the *Code of Ethics and Practice for Counsellors* (BAC, 1996a) that 'it is a breach of the ethical requirement for counsellors to practise without regular counselling supervision/consultative support'. Furthermore, the *Code of Ethics and Practice for Supervisors of Counsellors* (BAC, 1996b) states:

Counselling supervision is a formal and mutually agreed arrangement for counsellors to discuss their work regularly with someone who is normally an experienced and competent counsellor and familiar with the process of counselling supervision. The task is to work together to ensure and develop the efficacy of the supervisee's counselling practice.

I have included these extracts from counselling codes of practice because I feel they are appropriate for others in caring professions. The skills and the relevant theory are just as important in supporting the nurse supporting the patient and family as they are in counselling supervision.

The client–counsellor–supervisor relationship has many similarities to the patient (or parent)–nurse–supervisor (counsellor or mentor relationship). There is also the triad of the nurse–ward sister–supervisor/counsellor and the equivalent in the medical staff grading. Winnicott (1958) wrote extensively about the new mother needing to be emotionally held while she holds the baby, and recognised her need to be believed in as a 'good enough mother'. After many years in the nursing profession, I know that nurses need 'holding' themselves while they 'hold' the patient (and their family). They also need reassurance and encouragement to believe in themselves as a 'good enough' nurse.

Each person's need for support varies and must be respected. The more experienced ones may have developed their own coping strategies and know where to turn for advice or someone to talk to. For some, home and family, where the responsibilities and activities are totally different from work, make a necessary buffer for the pressures. For others, this is not possible, and help may be needed to identify the boundaries and limits of work in order to recognise the importance of 'time for me'. In a profession such as nursing and social work, it is very easy to become too involved, almost to the extent of feeling possessive about 'your' patient. This and other personal issues about work are often helped by talking in confidence to someone who understands.

Support needs to be ongoing for any individual. There is often a resistance to seeking help, especially amongst more senior staff and medical staff; some may see it as a weakness or failure. I would suggest that it should be a sign of strength to be taking positive action to help oneself. In my own experience of talking with medical students, they have welcomed the chance of talking in confidence to someone who is there to listen to them, and who understands the world of sick children and their families and the problems of the professionals. They express their feelings and their real fears of having to deliver bad news to parents, of witnessing their first death and how they will be expected to cope.

There may be feelings of failure, or that you performed less than perfectly, if you have not been able make a child better. I remind nurses of Winnicott's phrase – 'good enough mother' – and that they should take satisfaction from being a 'good enough' nurse. Winnicott added that perfection belongs to machines, not people.

A counselling role can assist individuals in their self-awareness and their observations of reactions in themselves and within a group. Clashes of personalities arise in any group, but in a working area such as this, it benefits everyone if difficulties can be worked through before they become disruptive. There is often a need to share personal feelings with someone or to 'dump' unwanted bad feeling in confidence.

It is not only work-related issues that can make life difficult at work. Personal worries and problems stay with us and are likely to affect our approach to work. Having someone to whom we can go and who will listen enables us to work through the difficulties. Quite often it is too costly, in both time and money, for individuals to seek professional help privately, so it becomes much more efficient to have someone available. It may well be that the person needing help should be advised to see their general practitioner, advice centre or appropriate agency. It may also be helpful to explore other possibilities such as aromatherapy, relaxation techniques, massage, and exercise classes or sports facilities.

SUPPORT GROUPS

Staff support groups meet regularly in some units, offering a forum for sharing work issues. Other units may have an understanding that time will be given as and when issues arise, as nurses must have someone to turn to if they wish, so they are not forced into bearing their burdens alone. There may be relief in discovering that a colleague has similar feelings about something: 'I thought it was just me, I'm glad I'm not the only one.' Peer support can offer much needed praise, encouragement, admiration and respect for a task done well – if group members are willing to give and to receive it.

When a group is formed, it is advisable to establish a few 'ground rules' at the start. The facilitator leads the group members in thinking about the purpose of the group: who will attend, where the group will meet, the frequency of meetings, dates and times of starting and finishing.

One of the most important issues is usually that of *confidentiality* – reassurance that whatever is said in the group, by anyone, will not be repeated outside the group. Without this guarantee, individuals will not feel safe to share their thoughts and feelings with others. The rules of confidentiality that protect the patients and families still apply in the group.

Other words to establish are *honesty* and *respect* – for the group rules, for each other, for what each has to say – allowing the person speaking to finish without being interrupted. Each person is in the group because he or she chooses to be and they all have as much right to be there as everyone else – they all belong.

A group might meet after a particular event, such as a death or traumatic incident, in order to share experiences with others who were there. The value of having an established staff support group which meets regularly is that when there is an urgent need for support, there is already a familiar 'place to go', and people are used to sharing and using the group. The support group should be held during work time, as staff are more likely to attend. It is seen to be valued support for the work when it is provided within the work setting, but group support should not be enforced.

Defusing

This is an informal intervention held after an event or period that has been particularly stressful for those involved. It may be quite simply a brief time to talk about what happened '...to make the incident less harmful. This is achieved by helping to restore control and by providing immediate assistance. It should reduce tension, focus on strengths and help carers to regain emotional control' (Wright, 1991).

Debriefing

After some traumatic events or distressing incidents, it is helpful to offer a more formal chance to debrief. Staff who were involved in the incident are helped to work through their memories and feelings, to prevent them also becoming victims of a disaster and to reduce the risk of developing post-traumatic stress disorder. Symptoms may include intrusive thoughts and dreams, repeated re-experiencing of emotions and sensations, avoidance of anything that might remind them of the incident, anxiety, shaking, depression and reluctance to go to work or to go home.

Wright (1991) reported, from studies of staff witnessing painful or traumatic events, that many suffered; one study concluded that staff counsellors should be available for everyday hospital events that cause stress, not only for disasters. I would agree, as I know that staff are faced with an enormous amount of stress and pressure, which when combined with what they give of themselves, both physically and emotionally, is a recipe for 'burn-out'. Important elements in any defusing or debriefing are strengthening of workers' coping skills, praise and thanks for a job well done, and permission to let go and move on.

Parkinson (1995) summarised the intention of debriefing as being to reduce the level of any possible symptoms at the time and later, and to reduce the possibility of the development of post-traumatic stress disorder. He advised the skilled debriefer to work through the process, either one-to-one or in a group, with the following guidelines:

1. Introduction – explaining the purpose and the process
2. The facts – participants' experiences, thoughts and impressions before the incident happened:
   — What were you doing?
   — Who were you with?
   — What were you talking about?
   — What was happening around you?
   — What were you thinking?
   — When were you aware that something was wrong or about to happen?
3. The feelings
   — sensory impressions (sights, sounds, smells, taste, touch)
   — feelings and emotions before, during and after the incident
4. The future – what resources are available to help?

SUPERVISION

Clinical supervision is being set up to be available for all nurses as 'an exchange between practising professionals to enable the development of professional skills' (Butterworth and Faugier, 1992). It is supportive in that 'by working with another person, the nurse can learn to become less personally overwhelmed by errors and to become analytical rather than emotional when dealing with them and then moving forward' (Hooton, 1994).

If we return to the role of supervision in counselling we find much of value for all health professionals. Carroll (1996) listed seven generic tasks of supervision:

- to set up a 'learning relationship'
- to teach
- to counsel
- to monitor professional ethical issues
- to evaluate
- to consult
- to monitor administrative aspects.

BAC (1996b) describes the nature of counselling supervision; a few points are reprinted here:

• Counselling supervision provides supervisees with the opportunity on a regular basis to discuss and monitor their work with clients. It should take account of the setting in which supervisees practise ... is intended to ensure that the needs of clients are being addressed and to monitor the effectiveness of the therapeutic interventions.

• ... supervision may contain some elements of training, personal development or line management, but counselling supervision is not primarily for these purposes and appropriate management of these issues should be observed.

• ... supervision is a formal collaborative process intended to help supervisees maintain ethical and professional standards of practice and to enhance creativity.

• It is important that counsellor and supervisor are able to work together constructively as counselling supervision includes supportive and challenging elements.

Supervision may be as an individual or in a group.

Appraisals

Regular appraisals for all members of staff are useful opportunities to reflect on individuals' own work and how they work with the team. A manager or team leader with good counselling skills will encourage feelings to be expressed and an honest discussion about how a role is developing, career progress and areas needing improvement. Most carers will remember only the criticism, so it is important to include praise for good skills and tasks well done.

A good appraisal will encourage the staff member to consider what has been learned in the context of the job and to think about future learning and training.

CONCLUSION

Working with sick children and their families is indeed stressful and everyone involved needs to learn their own ways of achieving a healthy and manageable balance between work and recreation, learning, reflecting on work practices, supporting others and ensuring support for themselves.

I would like to finish this chapter with a quote from Hawkins and Shohet (1989):

> There is so much pain and hurt in the world that, if we get caught into believing we have to make it better heroically; we are setting ourselves up to be overwhelmed and to burn out quickly. However, if we react to this reality with professional defensiveness, we may treat the symptoms, but we fail to meet and support the human beings who are communicating through these symptoms. The middle ground entails being on the path of facing our own shadow, our own fear, hurt and distress, and taking responsibility for ensuring that we practise what we preach. This means managing our own support system, finding friends and colleagues who will not just reassure us but also challenge our defences, and finding a supervisor or supervision group who ... will attend to how we are stuck in relating to the full truth of those with whom we work.

All of us working in the helping professions are human and we therefore cannot escape vulnerability to basic human emotions from within ourselves and from those we aim to help.

REFERENCES

British Association for Counselling (1996a) *Code of Ethics and Practice for Counsellors*. Rugby: BAC.

British Association for Counselling (1996b) *Code of Ethics and Practice for Supervisors of Counsellors*. Rugby: BAC.

Burnard, P. (1990) 'Stating the case.' Transcript of address: Project 2000 Interpersonal Skills in Nurse Training. *Counselling*, **1(4)**, 114–116.

Burnard, P. (1991) *Coping with Stress in the Health Professions*. London: Chapman and Hall.

Butterworth, C. & Faugier, J. (1992) *Clinical Supervision and Mentorship in Nursing*. London: Chapman and Hall.

Carroll, M. (1996) *Counselling Supervision*. London: Cassell.

Colville, G. (1998) Psychological support on the paediatric intensive care unit: a UK survey. *Care of the Critically Ill*, **14(1)**, 25–28.

Cook, P. (1993) The value of family counselling in paediatric intensive care. Abstracts from The Paediatric Intensive Care Society Spring Meeting, March 1993. *Care of the Critically Ill*, **9(4)**, 179.

Curran, A., Brighton, J. & Murphy, V. (1997) Psychoemotional care of parents of children in a neonatal intensive care unit: results of a questionaire. *Journal of Neonatal Nursing*, **3(1)**, 25–29.

Harding, R. (1996) Children with cancer: managing the staff. *Paediatric Nursing*, **8(3)**, 28–30.

Hawkins, P. & Shohet, R. (1989) *Supervision in the Helping Professions*. Milton Keynes: Open University Press.

Hooton, M. (1994) Clinical supervision. *Paediatric Nursing*, **6(7)**, 8–10.
Jolley, S. (1995) Nursing and stressful environments. *Paediatric Nursing*, 7(5), 28–29.
Jourard, S. (1971) *The Transparent Self*. New York: Van Nostrand Reinhold Co.
Jung, C. (1933) *Modern Man in Search of a Soul*. London: Ark Paperbacks, Routledge.
Lewis, C. (1998) Loss and change on the neonatal intensive care unit. *Paediatric Nursing*, **10(3)**, 21–23.
Menzies-Lyth, I. (1959) The functioning of social systems as a defence against anxiety. In *Containing Anxiety in Institutions*. London: Free Association Books.
National Association for Staff Support (1992) *A Charter for Staff Support – for Staff in the Health Care Services*. Woking: National Association for Staff Support.
Parkinson, F. (1995) Critical incident debriefing. *Counselling*, **6(3)**, 186–187.
Wesson, J. (1997) Meeting the informational, psychosocial and emotional needs of each ICU patient and family. *Intensive and Critical Care Nursing*, **13**, 111–118.
Winnicott, D. (1958) *Collected Papers: through Paediatrics to Psycho-analysis*. London: Tavistock Publications.
Winnicott, D. (1986) *Home is Where We Start From*. London: Penguin.
Wright, B. (1986) *Caring in Crisis – a Handbook of Intervention Skills for Nurses*. Edinburgh: Churchill Livingstone.
Wright, B. (1991) *Sudden Death – Intervention Skills for the Caring Professions*. Edinburgh: Churchill Livingstone.

Conclusion

It does not seem quite right to call the final words of this book a 'conclusion' since there will be no end to discussions such as these. The support of sick children and their families may involve many professional roles, a huge range of illnesses and conditions, long-term or short-term care and emergency and crisis interventions. In this book, I have tried to explore some of these issues. I hope you find them helpful, interesting and relevant to your own work with families.

I have made a considerable number of references to the writings of others when it felt appropriate. It is definitely not an exhaustive list of references so there is plenty of scope, for those of you with more time than I have, to conduct your own more detailed literature searches. I have mentioned already the value of teamwork; somehow there is a feeling of being united as a team with the thoughts of others on the same issues.

The order of the chapters is not particularly significant. Those concerned with feelings and emotions are an essential part of all the others. I think they are particularly important for staff to think about in relation to how they view the children and families in their care. Otherwise they may label the parents 'awkward' or the child 'difficult' and then no one benefits. Wright (1986) said, most appropriately: 'We cannot be part of the healing process and ignore the psychological problems; our need to respond to these problems is as great as the patient's need for them to be met.'

Each of us may respond differently to the situations we face. This does not mean that any person is wrong. It does not imply weakness to share concerns and feelings with colleagues. Counselling skills are not magical powers bestowed on a few; they are present in most people who choose to work in the caring professions, otherwise they would not continue to do this work. The skills can be learnt and staff may need to refresh them regularly, by reading or attending workshops; they are valuable tools for coping and helping with some degree of confidence. Sometimes there does not seem to be anything to say or do to help, only to acknowledge and listen.

Professionals should always be able to feel supported in whatever way they need; the work is not easy and shows no sign of becoming any easier! But life for families of sick children is not easy either. Most parents care for their children adequately if not well. It is, however, a tragic fact that this is not so for all families, and for me, one of the saddest truths about working in paediatrics is that some children do not deserve the parents to whom they have had the misfortune to be born. Good teamwork between those who help and those who are being helped is essential to the well-being of both parties.

At the end of the day, or when you are feeling you have no more to give, perhaps you can allow yourself to accept that the problems of other people are not necessarily your problems. You are fortunate enough to be able to leave them, but perhaps with the reassurance that you did what you could to support sick children and their families.

REFERENCE

Wright, B. (1986) *Caring in Crisis – a Handbook of Intervention Skills for Nurses.* Edinburgh: Churchill Livingstone.

Appendix: Useful addresses, contacts and telephone numbers

Action for Sick Children
300 Kingston Road, Wimbledon Chase, London SW20 8LX
Tel: 0181 542 4848
Fax: 0181 542 2424

'Being Yourself'
(Books, therapeutic games and materials for professionals and children)

Deal, Kent CT1A 7NN
Tel: 01304 381333

British Association for Counselling
1 Regent Place, Rugby, Warwickshire CV21 2PJ
Tel: 01788 578328 (information) Fax: 01788 562189
    01788 550899 (office) Minicom: 01788 572828

British Organ Donor Society (BODY)
Balsham, Cambridge CB1 6DL
(Offers help and support to donor and recipient families, as well as promoting organ donation and transplantation)

Tel: 01223 893636

CADD (Campaign Against Drink Driving)
83 Jesmond Road, Newcastle upon Tyne NE2 1NH
Tel: 0191 281 1581

Child Accident Prevention Trust
18–20 Farringdon Lane, London EC1R 3AU

The Child Bereavement Trust
(Supports professionals through training and resources)

Brindley House, 4 Burkes Road, Beaconsfield, Bucks HP9 1PB (liable to alteration)
Tel/Fax: 01628 488101

Child Death Helpline
(Staffed by bereaved parents for anyone affected by the death of a child. Every evening 7–10 p.m. and Wednesdays 10 a.m.–1 p.m.)

Freephone: 0800 282986

Childrens' Head Injury Trust
c/o Neurosurgery Dept, The Radcliffe Infirmary,
Woodstock Road, Oxford OX2 6HE
Tel: 01865 224786

The Compassionate Friends
(*A nationwide and international organisation for bereaved parents, by bereaved parents*)

53, North Street, Bristol BS3 1EN
Tel: 0117 9665202
Helpline: 0117 9539639

Contact-a-Family
170 Tottenham Court Road, London W1P 0HA
Tel: 0171 383 3555 (contact line)

Cot Death Helpline
Tel: 0171 235 1721 (24 hours/day)

CRUSE Bereavement Care
(*The largest bereavement care organisation offering help to all bereaved people – advice and counselling, groups and social events, training courses for volunteers and health care professionals, and many publications*)

126 Sheen Road, Richmond, Surrey TW9 1UR
Tel: 0181 9404818 Helpline: 0181 3327227

Foundation for the Study of Infant Deaths
14 Halkin Street, London SW1X 7DP
Tel: 0171 235 0965
Fax: 0171 823 1986

National Association of Bereavement Services
(*Puts bereaved in touch with local services and offers telephone counselling and advice*)

20 Norton Folgate, London E1 6BD
Tel: 0171 247 0617
Helpline: 0171 247 1080

React
(*Research, Education and Aid for Children with Potentially Terminal Illness*)

St Luke's House, 270 Sandycombe Road, Kew, Richmond, Surrey TW9 3NP
Tel: 0181 940 2575
Fax: 0181 940 2050

Relate
(*See local telephone directory*)

Tel: 01788 563816

Resources
Meditec Medical and Nursing Booksellers
Jackson's Yard, Brewery Hill, Grantham, Lincs NG31 6DW
Tel: 01476 590505
Fax: 01476 590329

RoadPeace
(National charity supporting road traffic victims)

PO Box 2579, London NW10 3PW
Tel: 0181 964 9353

SANDS (Stillbirth and Neonatal Death Society
Argyle House, 29–31 Euston Road, London NW1 2SD
Tel: 0171 436 5881 (weekdays 10 a.m.–5 p.m.)

The Sick Children's Trust
(Supporting families with sick children)

1A Doughty Street, London WC1N 2PH
Tel: 0171 404 3329
Fax: 0171 831 3182

Victim Support
(See local telephone directory)

Victim Support (England, Wales and Northern Ireland)
Cranmer House, 39 Brixton Road, London SW9 6DZ
Tel: 0171 735 9166

Victim Support (Scotland)
14 Frederick Street, Edinburgh EH2 2HB
Tel: 0131 225 7779

Index